Narrative Medicine
in Hospice Care

Studies in the Thought of Paul Ricoeur

Series Editors
Greg S. Johnson, Pacific Lutheran University/Oxford University (ELAC)
Dan R. Stiver, Hardin-Simmons University

Studies in the Thought of Paul Ricoeur, a series in conjunction with the Society for Ricoeur Studies, aims to generate research on Ricoeur, about whom interest is rapidly growing both nationally (United States and Canada) and internationally. Broadly construed, the series has three interrelated themes. First, we develop the historical connections to and in Ricoeur's thought. Second, we extend Ricoeur's dialogue with contemporary thinkers representing a variety of disciplines. Third, we utilize Ricoeur to address future prospects in philosophy and other fields that respond to emerging issues of importance. The series approaches these themes from the belief that Ricoeur's thought is not just suited to theoretical exchanges, but can and does matter for how we actually engage in the many dimensions that constitute lived existence.

Recent Titles in the Series

A Companion to Ricoeur's Fallible Man,
edited by Scott Davidson

Ricoeur's Hermeneutics of Religion:
Rebirth of the Capable Self,
by Brian Gregor

Ideology and Utopia in the Twenty-first Century:
The Surplus of Meaning in Ricoeur's Dialectical Concept,
edited by Stephanie Arel and Dan R. Stiver

Ricoeur and the Third Discourse of the Person:
From Philosophy and Neuroscience to Psychiatry and Theology,
by Michael T. H. Wong

A Companion to Ricoeur's Freedom and Nature,
edited by Scott Davidson

Paul Ricoeur's Moral Anthropology:
Singularity, Responsibility, and Justice,
by Geoffrey Dierckxsens

Narrative Medicine in Hospice Care

Identity, Practice, and Ethics through the Lens of Paul Ricoeur

Tara Flanagan

LEXINGTON BOOKS
Lanham • Boulder • New York • London

Published by Lexington Books
An imprint of The Rowman & Littlefield Publishing Group, Inc.
4501 Forbes Boulevard, Suite 200, Lanham, Maryland 20706
www.rowman.com

6 Tinworth Street, London SE11 5AL, United Kingdom

Copyright © 2020 by The Rowman & Littlefield Publishing Group, Inc.

All rights reserved. No part of this book may be reproduced in any form or by any electronic or mechanical means, including information storage and retrieval systems, without written permission from the publisher, except by a reviewer who may quote passages in a review.

British Library Cataloguing in Publication Information Available

Library of Congress Cataloging-in-Publication Data Available

ISBN 978-1-4985-5462-6 (cloth)
ISBN 978-1-4985-5464-0 (pbk)
ISBN 978-1-4985-5463-3 (electronic)

Contents

Acknowledgments   vii

Introduction   ix

1 Narrative Medicine: The Turn toward Narrative in Clinical Practice   1

2 Narrative Identity and Practice in the Hospice Model of Care   31

3 Narrative Ethics and Practices from the Patient's Perspective: Life Review as Ethical Self-Assessment   59

4 The Limits of Narrative Medicine for End-of-Life Patients   83

5 Expanding beyond Narrative: Hospitality, Accompaniment, and Companioning as Models of Presence with Patients   107

Bibliography   127

Index   139

About the Author   145

Acknowledgments

My mentor at Loyola University Chicago, Hille Haker, brought boundless enthusiasm, insight, and dedication to this research. Every time I would meet with her one-on-one, I would leave the encounter awed by her perception, encyclopedic knowledge, and thoughtful commentary. I am deeply indebted to her for sharing her time and vision with me.

Many faculty members at Loyola served as figures of academic support and personal encouragement during my time in Chicago, particularly Jon Nilson, Sandra Sullivan-Dunbar, Edmondo Lupieri, Mark Waymack, and Susan Ross, Chair of the Department of Theology and Religious Studies at the time. Special thanks to Loyola University Chicago librarian, Jane Currie, subject specialist in theology and religious studies, who truly went above and beyond in the level of support, expertise, and guidance she provided, as well as to Jennifer Stegen, the interlibrary loan coordinator. Completing my research would not have been possible without the financial support provided by the graduate school at Loyola University Chicago and the research funding provided by the Arthur J. Schmitt Foundation.

Scholars at the Midwest Regional American Academy of religion gave me opportunities to present and develop my research on narrative medicine, religion, and ethics on many occasions. I am particularly indebted to Jason Mahn who heard an earlier paper I presented on narrative medicine and provided thoughtful feedback during the session. His compassionate insight informed a great deal of my research, and I am grateful for his intellectual generosity and kindness.

Dr. Haker coordinated monthly research seminars, always lively and stimulating, where I benefited from the feedback of John Crowley-Buck, Christian Cintron, Dan Dion, Grant Gholson, Michael McCarthy, Silas Morgan, Erica Saccucci, and Sara Wilhelm Garbers. Thank you as well to Trevor Clark,

Kevin Considine, Lauren O'Connell, Jeanine Viau, Andrea Hollingsworth, and Jesse Perillo for your enriching company. Due to Dr. Haker's commitment to interdisciplinary collaboration across borders, I had the opportunity to meet and learn from faculty and students at Erfurt University, particularly Christof Mandry, Henning Bühmann, and Gwendolin Wanderer. A conference held at Goethe University in Frankfurt allowed me to collaborate with chaplains and scholars of religion and medicine and to present and develop this research further.

At Maria College, I am incredibly grateful to Sr. Victoria Battell, Peter Byrne, Anne Devlin, Thomas Gamble, and Anne Jung for your support and gracious welcome to the Maria community. Thank you as well to my students for our time together and for your dedication to learning and service.

I have deep gratitude for Dan Stiver and Greg Johnson, both for their feedback and for including this book in their series on the work of Paul Ricoeur. Thank you to Kenneth Reynhout, from the American Academy of Religion Ricoeur group, who encouraged me to develop and publish this research. Special thanks to those at Lexington Books, particularly Jana Hodges-Kluck and Sydney Wedbush for their guidance on the manuscript and for shepherding me through the review process.

My heartfelt gratitude to John Tracy and Tom and Kathryn Tracy for their unfailing support along the way. Thank you also to Bob and Tamara Odell for your hospitality and kindness. I am grateful for the buoyant presence of William Tracy, who encouraged me to take breaks to play and go outside, and for the sense of wonder he brings to my world.

Finally, I would like to thank the hospice clinicians, caregivers, volunteers, family members, and patients that I was privileged to meet during my work with hospice. It was an honor and blessing to be in your presence.

Introduction

Clinical encounters between caregivers and patients can be reciprocally rewarding, with an atmosphere of understanding and a sense of being seen and heard developing between a patient—a person fundamentally in need of care—and a caregiver there to listen to and treat the patient's concerns. There are few places where one can openly discuss one's vulnerabilities and fears, but clinical environments such as the doctor's office or a hospital room, counterintuitively, provide a space where one can freely discuss the limits of the body and the existential concerns provoked by these limits. While the clinical encounter can be deepened through intimate conversation on a personal level, in clinical education the communication skills needed to engage in such dialogue are prioritized less than physical care for the body, a biological reductionism that leaves clinicians and patients alike craving a more meaningful, personal interaction. The field of narrative medicine developed in response to the desire of clinicians to cultivate their skills in attentive listening and close attention to the interpretations of embodiment provided by patients.[1] Narrative medicine originated as a practice of care intended for physicians, but has since expanded to include other clinical caregiving professions such as chaplaincy, social work, and other clinicians dedicated to therapeutic patient care.

This book examines practices of narrative medicine and moral identity for end-of-life patients with special attention given to the work of Paul Ricoeur, particularly the work of Ricoeur's that addresses patient identity and healthcare ethics. Narrative medicine is a mode of clinical practice structured on the belief that a close reading of literature can sharpen a clinician's ability to attend to patients in the clinical encounter. Additionally, patients themselves find opportunities for expression and processing their experience in health care through narrative practices. In this text, I examine modalities of narrative practice for both clinicians and patients. However, I also take into account those patients who are unable to engage in dialogue with their caregivers due to verbal or cognitive limits. While noting the genuine value of narrative medicine for clinicians, I examine the limits of self-narration for patients who are unable to offer a linear, coherent narrative of their lives due to cognitive deficits such as Alzheimer's disease. For patients so challenged, I suggest that the concept of patient identity and the practices of caregiving described by Paul Ricoeur and Cicely Saunders transcend the need for higher-level cognition commonly associated with narrative medicine. Throughout the text, I demonstrate how the hospice model of care recognizes both the value and the limits of a narrative practices as they apply to end-of-life patients and provides a treatment model for patients regardless of their verbal and cognitive abilities.

Paul Ricoeur, whose work on hermeneutical phenomenology represents a cross-pollination of philosophy, theology, and ethics, offers a perspective on narrative identity that expands beyond the models of selfhood presumed in narrative medicine. For Ricoeur, identity is shaped by the tensions between continuity and change, facticity and invention, relatedness and singularity, and certainty and mystery. As he states in *Oneself as Another*, though we might like to think we are the hero of our own narrative, with inward awareness of our motivations and goals, there are dimensions of one's own selfhood that are fundamentally unknowable.[2] Ricoeur's work on narrative identity offers a needed expansion on the one assumed in the medical model, one which bears the imprint of Aristotle's view of narrativity as presented in the *Poetics*. Ricoeur's work is particularly relevant for clinicians providing care to patients who are nonverbal or patients with limited cognitive capacities, such as those with dementia. My purpose in this book is to show how Ricoeur's view of narrative selfhood can serve as a resource for clinicians trained in narrative medicine, particularly those who may find themselves unprepared or uncomfortable working with patients with limited verbal capacities.

In chapter 1, I address the reforms in medical education, which resulted in restructuring the pedagogical model in the United States from one based on the healing arts to one based on biology, chemistry, and a laboratory model of education. This shift enhanced clinical care for the treatment of the patient's body and created space for the field of evidence-based medical research. However, this turn toward science, or biological positivism, in medicine, combined with an approach to medicine based on clinical detachment, left many patients and clinicians feeling dissatisfied with medical treatment. The patient's experience as an embodied individual in need of recognition and tailored care became secondary, supplanted by a standardized model of clinical care for the body. What Paul Ricoeur and the practitioner-scholars in narrative medicine have to offer is a retrieval of the patient's experience as a valuable source of information and connection in the clinical encounter. Through narrative practices of clinical care, the patient, and the patient's interpretation of the illness experience, offered to and heard by their caregiver, health care can move toward a more balanced model of evidence-based medicine and person-centered care.

Chapter 2 outlines the concept of patient identity as it exists in the hospice model of care with specific attention given to Cicely Saunders's perspective on the many dimensions of pain for patients at the end of life. Saunders, trained as a nurse, social worker, and physician, and the founder of St. Christopher's Hospice in 1967, recognized that the patients she worked with experienced more than just physical pain. From her conversations with patients over the years, she learned from her patients that their distress was also personal, social, and existential in nature. Because of her advocacy for comprehensive pain management, hospice medical teams now include social workers, chaplains, bereavement counselors, and volunteers who are available to address a patient's needs beyond physical pain management. The definition of pain I use, "total pain," is defined by Cicely Saunders as physical, spiritual, existential, and psychosocial pain. In this chapter, I describe the ways in which religious and spiritual care serves a needed role in the care of end-of-life patients, noting the role chaplains and physicians play in addressing the religious and spiritual dimensions of patient experience.

In chapter 3, I examine a specific form of narrative practice called life review, a model of retrospective self-reflection patients may engage in when facing the end of life. I describe the ways in which life review represents a form of ethical self-reflection in which a patient evaluates how one's life was lived. Patients can experience regret, grief over lost time, and a desire for forgiveness—all themes that suggest self-evaluation. Life review is a common narrative-based intervention for healthcare chaplains, and chaplains are available to address the spiritual pain that can emerge during life review as the themes of regret, grief, and a desire for forgiveness are manifestations of emotional pain that have a spiritual or religious valence. Although physical pain is located in the body and can often be treated pharmacologically, spiritual pain has various sources and calls for specialized attention. Professional chaplains serve on hospice interdisciplinary teams to address these needs which can become acute as death nears.

Because a chaplain is not usually at an admission or present in an initial clinical encounter, it is crucial that the admitting clinician is familiar with how to take a spiritual assessment, another dialogical clinical practice, and feels comfortable making a chaplain referral to address a patient's spiritual care needs. Patients commonly structure their end-of-life treatment decisions on their religious views.[3] In *Theological Bioethics*, Lisa Cahill suggests that the role of the religious dimension of human experience needs to be revisited in medical care:

> [T]he practice of medicine and the provision of health care are in our culture increasingly scientific rather than humanistic enterprises, and they are even more quickly being directed by marketplace values. Participants in biomedicine—whether providers or patients—are finding this situation ever less satisfactory at a personal level, and many are raising questions about the kind of society that is sponsoring these shifts, in turn to be re-created by them. Because they deal in the elemental human experiences of birth, life, death, and suffering, the biomedical arts provide an opening for larger questions of meaning or even of transcendence. Religious themes and imagery can be helpful in articulating these concerns and addressing them in an imaginative, provocative, and perhaps ultimately transformative way.[4]

The end of life brings questions of meaning, identity, and moral behavior into sharp relief. Therefore, the need for clinicians to be comfortable with religiosity and spirituality when demonstrated by their patients is even higher for those receiving hospice and palliative care than it is for those receiving standard clinical care. As religion is linked closely to conceptions of the moral self on the part of the patient, to overlook the role of religiosity in a patient's life is to neglect an important source of clinical information.

I turn in chapter 4 to the limits of narrative medicine, taking into account limits due to patient's capacities to engage verbally as well as the limits that come from a patient's context of care. In this chapter, I address cognitive decline in end-of-life patients and address the impediments to verbal ability that can come with such decline, leading to unintelligible speech. The literature on narrative medicine depends a great deal on a concept of the self as narrating agent. In chapter 4, I supplement this concept by describing elements of narrative selfhood that are marked by discontinuity and fragmentation. I identify levels of narrativity for patients and speak to the ways narrative concepts of patient identity can be understood as social, rather than just originating with individual patients. Ricoeur's view of social selfhood proves useful when taking into account patients who are unable to offer their own narrative understanding of their lives due to cognitive or verbal constraints.

In chapter 5, I consider modes of presence with patients that expand beyond narrative-based practices. I address the ways clinicians can attend to patients with compromised verbal and cognitive abilities, specifically through models of presence that do not rely on any capacity on the patient's part, such as the ability to engage in reciprocal dialogue. I maintain that the Christian practice of hospitality in the form of welcoming the stranger holds particular value for clinicians engaging with patients who have limited neurological or verbal capacity. Religious approaches to patient care also allow for a way of viewing patients that does not rely on their ability to speak or respond to the clinician. I examine the contributions of Paul

Ricoeur's view of accompaniment as a nonnarrative based form of presence with the dying and the theologically informed practice of hospitality as they relate to working with this population of patients. I identify a selection of nonverbal forms of religious and spiritual presence that can enhance care for end-of-life patients, particularly with regard to a patient's social needs. The modes of presence that I speak to are options for both clinical caregivers and nonclinical caregivers.

Managing physical pain is a priority in medical care and rightly so. My concern in this work is neglect of the other dimensions of patients' pain:

1. Social isolation and loneliness of the elderly and dying
2. Psychosocial and spiritual distress as a manifestation of total pain

Patients who are not pleasurable or rewarding to visit, such as those with dementia or those who are angry or in moral distress as a result of life review, can go unvisited and unattended to because they are challenging to be with. They do not provide the reciprocity that is celebrated in narrative medicine, which has focused up to this point on verbal, coherent patients. Drawing on the Matthean understanding of the vulnerable and marginalized, I see these patients as "the least of these," the hungry, thirsty, naked, sick, and imprisoned—the stranger; those that, in a medical field focused on health and healing, may have inward pain that goes unrecognized. My central question is this: What does care for the least of these mean for those at the end of life? Whose care might be overlooked when it comes to comprehensive pain management, care that goes beyond physical, bodily pain? Hospice offers an expanded concept of pain that includes, but expands beyond, the narrow view of pain as a physical state of being. I look to hospice as a model for the treatment of pain in its myriad forms as a model for practicing hospitality and the corporal works of mercy.

From an ethics perspective, my goal in this book is to consider those patients who go unvisited and those who fall outside of the patient population considered in current models of narrative medicine. I examine the complications of approaching the clinical encounter with the expectation that the patient will offer stimulating dialogue or dialogical reciprocity. Patients are often anxious, confused, suspicious, or in pain. Such patients, even when capable of engaging in dialogue with their clinicians, may not have the energy or desire to engage in conversation about their concerns beyond their immediate experience. Many patients, especially those at the end of life, are unable to offer a verbal response to caregivers and the needs of these patients can go unaddressed in narrative medicine as it exists currently. My primary goal is to bring attention to patients that may present as challenging for clinicians due to reasons related to physical, personal, social, and existential pain that affect patient behavior or due to the verbal or cognitive limits of patients who are unable to offer a narrative account of their experience. The features of identity highlighted by Ricoeur—our fragility, vulnerability, and interrelatedness—offer a needed expansion on the concepts of patient identity that are limited to the body or even to narrative capacities. In *Oneself as Another*, and in his posthumously published collection, *Living Up to Death*, Ricoeur, like Saunders, recognizes the need to attend to the personal, social, spiritual, and existential dimensions of human experience, a perspective that supplements concepts of patient identity in the biomedical model of care.[5]

NOTES

1. The term "narrative medicine" was coined by literature scholar and physician, Rita Charon, who founded and directs a clinical program on narrative medicine for physicians and other health-care providers. Her text *Narrative Medicine: Honoring the Stories of Illness* (Oxford University Press, 2006) and the co-authored text *Principles and Practice of Narrative Medicine* (Oxford University Press, 2017) provide details on methods used in practicing narrative medicine and the benefits of such practices.

2. Paul Ricoeur, *Oneself as Another*, trans. David Pellauer (Chicago, IL: University of Chicago Press, 1992).

3. Daniel Sulmasy, "Ethos, Mythos, and Thanatos: Spirituality and Ethics at the End of Life," *Journal of Pain and Symptom Management* 46, no. 3 (2013): 447–51.

4. Lisa Sowle Cahill, *Theological Bioethics: Participation, Justice, and Change* (Washington, DC: Georgetown University Press, 2005).

5. Paul Ricoeur, *Living Up to Death* (Chicago, IL: University of Chicago Press, 2009).

Chapter 1

Narrative Medicine

The Turn toward Narrative in Clinical Practice

Medical practitioners, including physicians, nurses, chaplains, and physical and mental health therapists, in the attempt to better their ability to provide care, have turned to the study of narrative to develop their clinical skills with patients and family members. Expanding beyond an efficiency-model of medicine, such practitioners are concerned with treating patients as individuals and deepening their ability to listen to patients as patients express their physical, psychosocial, and existential concerns. Additionally, patients themselves have turned to narrative methods to express their resistance to being treated as an object—as a body, a diagnosis, a subject of research or experimental treatments—detached from their personhood and history. In this chapter, I examine the history of medical care in the United States with the goal of tracing the turn toward narrative practices in medicine.

Following the release of the Flexner report in 1910, commissioned by the Carnegie Foundation under the aegis of the newly formed American Medical Association, medical education in the United States was intentionally restructured to become both more uniform across the country and more science-based.[1] Abraham Flexner, familiar with the German model of medical training in which physicians were trained as scientists, evaluated medical schools in the United States and Canada, judging them based on the education levels of practicing physicians and on the quality of their laboratory facilities.[2,3] In his report, which denounced many US hospitals as substandard, he recommended that medical education be amended to include laboratory training and research, moving toward a lab model of education rather than a lecture model of education. Research in cell biology, organic chemistry, and physiology were hallmarks of the German model, and, following the Flexner report—a catalyst for dramatic reform in medical education—these subjects were prioritized in the United States system as well.[4] The Flexner report is seen as the turning point in North American medical training, when medical education shifted from a focus on healing to a disease-based model focused on scientific research and curative treatment.

In addition to Abraham Flexner's role in medical education reform, the work of Morris Fishbein created momentum for the pivot toward the science-centered focus of clinical education that exists today. Editor of the *Journal of the American Medical Association* from 1924 to 1950, Fishbein, who shared Flexner's passion for reform in medical education, became committed to defining medicine as a scientific pursuit that required substantial education in what would later come to be called evidence-based medicine.[5] Wary of medical fads and "quacks," he worked to inspire an approach to medicine oriented to the role of the physician as medium: it was the science that cured the patient, not the doctor.[6] As a result, doctors qua scientists have "four fundamental tasks," based on problem-solving and research:

1. Finding out what is the matter (diagnosis)
2. Finding out how it happened (cause)
3. Deciding what to do (treatment)
4. Predicting the outcome (prognosis)[7]

Fishbein responded with indignance to homeopathic healers claiming to work under the purview of medicine, but lacking a foundation of clinical medical education, and using ethically and medically questionable treatment methods, famously, snake oil.[8] Fishbein's dedication to the professionalization of medicine, and the megaphone that came with his role as long-time editor of the *Journal of the American Medical Association,* played a major role in medical education reform. The momentum toward reform at the turn of the twentieth century culminated with the model of evidence-based medicine dominant in the United States today. The diagnosis-cause-treatment-prognosis model remains effective for meeting patient's acute medical needs, but the goals of care for other medical concerns, like chronic health conditions or terminal illnesses, do not necessarily fit a curative model. The turn toward narrative concepts of patient identity and clinical practice can be seen as a response to the efficient, yet mechanistic, treatment of patients, treatment that can result from a problem-solving, generalized model of care.

The reforms in medical education lead to the professionalization of medicine as a field marked by scientific rigor and high standards in clinical education. Yet, as medicine became systematized, patients began to feel overlooked or objectified, seen as experiments, body parts, or diseases, and scrutinized as objects of pathology. As early as 1910, patients were critiquing the detached impersonal care they received in hospitals.[9] Sophisticated care meant specialized, professional care, marked by a growing reliance on diagnostic technology, rather than on personalized care tailored to a patient's needs, experiences, and fears. What was perceived as impersonal care resulted from an institutional focus on administration, surgery, laboratory and X-ray tests, and methods of treatment that made the hospital a place for technology-based treatment rather than human encounter.[10] In some hospitals, patients were known by their bed number rather than their names—this was intentionally done to keep a professional, yet therapeutic, distance between the patients and nurses.[11] As a result of being treated as a body, a number, or a diagnosis, patients became dissatisfied with treatment in which they were not seen, heard, or recognized as a person. Consequently, patients voiced their critique through autobiographical illness narratives. Patients might have been receiving higher quality, more effective medical care, but their experience receiving this sophisticated clinical attention was perceived as impersonal and dehumanizing.

CLINICAL DETACHMENT AS A PRACTICAL SKILL FOR HEALTH CARE PROVIDERS

The expression "clinical detachment" arose during the 1950s when sociologists observed how medical students related to patients during their training.[12] Originally a descriptive term, "clinical detachment" has now become normative in the field, a stance a clinician intentionally cultivates, possibly to appear more professional, possibly to avoid compassion fatigue.[13] Research shows that the empathic regard for patients that medical students start their training with begins to decline as they progress in their studies.[14] Physician and poet Jack Coulehan identifies what he terms the "hidden curriculum" in medical schools as the possible culprit, a curriculum oriented to objectivity, suspicion of emotionality in patients and even oneself, and a focus on empirical and technical data, rather than patients' interpretations of their experience.

Coulehan suggests that there are three possible scenarios for a clinician's approach to care when they graduate: some leave as technicians, some leave with the empathic presence they came with, and a large group leaves with what he calls "non-reflective professionalism."[15] These clinicians are the ones that, over the course of their medical training, have become less compassionate and more emotionally detached from their patients, resulting from the hidden curriculum that teaches students that the objectivity that results from a posture of clinical detachment will allow one to provide better care for patients.[16] Clinicians with detached concern are not unfeeling, but they have learned to practice medicine with some distance from the world of the patient, particularly the symbolic, meaning-oriented world of the patient. It is this world of meaning, this inner world of experience, that interests those doing research and clinical practice based on narrative medicine. Their hope is to close the gap between clinician and patient, developing what Coulehan calls "clinical empathy" as part of the clinician's skill-set.[17] For physician-scholars like Rita Charon, who examines literature and medicine, and Christina Puchalski, whose scholarship addresses religion and medicine, the goal is also to have an explicit curriculum centered on the use of resources that work to cultivate empathic regard rather than detachment in the way clinicians respond to patients.[18]

Due to the emphasis on empirical methods in medical training and the intentional cultivation of clinical detachment in residents, it is understandable that patients experiencing a health crisis may come to feel alienated by the biomedical model of care, a model focused on research, technologized treatment, and emotional distance, rather than on empathic concern and personal connection. The proliferation of illness memoirs, a form of protest literature in which patients reclaim their personhood and individual experience in the institutional model of medicine, can be seen as a result of patients not feeling heard or validated by their clinicians. Sayantani DasGupta's *Stories of Illness and Healing* speaks to medical treatment as fundamentally inhumane, particularly for women. For disenfranchised patients, writing can be a way of reclaiming agency in a time of powerlessness.[19]

THE TURN TOWARD NARRATIVE IN THE MEDICAL HUMANITIES

Literature scholar Ann Jurecic named the AIDS epidemic in the 1980s as the cultural moment that led to the burgeoning genre of illness narratives, noting that there were few accounts of the global influenza epidemic of 1918/1919 in comparison. Though more lives were taken by the flu than US soldiers killed in World War I, and there were more deaths as a result of the flu in one year than there were from the Black Death over a century, there was very little written about it compared to the narrative accounts of those affected by the HIV.[20] Due to uncertainty about how one contracts the virus, and to the social stigma of AIDS as a "gay plague," activists responded by urging those infected to speak up about their diagnosis, recognizing that talking about AIDS would decrease the power of the taboo, lead to more funding for research, and possibly decrease infection rates. Activists used the catchphrase "Silence = Death" to urge people to speak about their disease in the hopes of modifying the public perception of the virus.[21]

Clinicians came to be seen in a negative light around the same time as the turn toward narrative in the medical humanities, particularly in autobiographical illness accounts. The concept of a physician as detached, cold, and heartless, even malicious, became a familiar theme in illness narratives, a binary being created between the innocent, vulnerable patient and the unfeeling, scientist doctor. When medical training transitioned from a healing model to a model based on the sciences, particularly chemistry and biology, the patient's experience moved from the foreground to the background.[22] Medical education in the United States developed into a type of "applied biology" as noted by philosopher and clinical ethicist Richard Zaner.[23] Patient narratives reveal that they felt unseen and unheard. Anne Hunsaker Hawkins sees a change in how medical testimonials changed over time. She notes that in the 1960s and 1970s patients' accounts were not necessarily critical of medical care and the medical system. However, testimonials in the 1980s had more of a decidedly angry, accusatory tone. She uses the language of "medically syntonic" and "medically dystonic" to describe the differences in patient accounts.[24] One could say that by the 1980s patients had decided that they would be the subject of medical treatment, rather than the object of medical treatment.

The proliferation of patient accounts coincides with academic interest in the clinical encounter. Michael Balint, inspired by Carl Rogers's dedication to "client-centered" therapy, used the language of "patient-centered" medicine in 1970.[25] The turn toward narrative in the humanities and social sciences, particularly the turn toward narrative in medical anthropology, can be traced to the publication of Clifford Geertz' *Interpretation of Cultures* in 1973,[26] and, more specifically, to the publication of Arthur Kleinman's text *The Illness Narratives: Suffering, Healing, and the Human Condition* in 1988.[27] Other notable figures in the history of narrative medicine include psychologist Jerome Bruner and his influential work on narrative selfhood. Bruner is famous for saying, "it is through narrative that we create and recreate selfhood," going so far as to say that selfhood requires the ability to narrate.[28] Published in 1977, George Engel's pioneering book on the biopsychosocial model of care also worked to draw attention to the limits of biological positivism in medicine and the need to approach a patient contextually, taking into account a patient's individual, psychological concerns.[29] Cheryl Mattingly's work on narrative reasoning in occupational therapy, and the work of medical anthropologists Byron Good and Mary Jo Delvecchio Good, examines the clinical encounter itself, analyzing it as an hermeneutical exchange worthy of critical analysis.[30]

Philosophers Alasdair MacIntyre and Paul Ricouer also contributed to the turn toward narrative in the humanities. MacIntyre, describing humans as the "story-telling animal," examines the ways narratives are used to as devices for individuals who need to reconcile their behavior with their ideal of selfhood.[31] In *After Virtue*, he links narrativity to the moral dimensions of selfhood, claiming virtue relies on the "concept of a self whose unity resides in the unity of a narrative which links birth to life to death as narrative beginning to middle to end."[32] Ricoeur emphasizes the imaginative, even fictitious, features of self-making, claiming that humans engage in a process of organizing and interpreting events in their lives in the attempt to achieve narrative unity. MacIntyre uses the language of "epistemological crises" to describe the conflict between a person's expectations and reality as they experience it. Narratives are then adapted to fit an individual's modified worldview.[33] Both MacIntyre and Ricoeur maintain that narrative selfhood involves both reflection on one's past self and projection about one's future self. Humans historicize their lives and then plot their lives intentionally, working toward chosen or possible life goals—Ricoeur uses the language of the kingdom of the "as if" to describe the realm of the possible.[34] Ricoeur's work on narrative identity, expanding beyond MacIntyre's, details the aspects of selfhood that fall outside of the neat lines of beginning, middle, and end. He also recognizes the dimensions of selfhood that are inaccessible to us or that are relational and narrated by others—elements of narrativity that an individual has limited control over.

The turn toward narrative in the medical humanities coincides with the development of formal bioethics and the focus on agency and autonomy in Beauchamp and Childress' principalist model of medical ethics.[35] Similarly, agency and autonomy, and their limits, are common themes in illness narratives, along with the persistent grievance that one's personhood is being neglected in medical care. With regard to bioethics, details about the inhumane treatment of medical research subjects cast a spotlight on the objectification and dehumanization of patients, leading to the formal recognition of medical ethics and patient rights in the *Belmont Report*, written in 1978.[36] Figures such as Peter Buxtun, whistleblower on the Tuskegee syphilis experiment, called attention to how those in need of medical care were surreptitiously being used to further medical research rather than receiving medical treatment.[37] Even the title of Paul Ramsey's classic text *Patient as Person* captures the sense that the patient was being objectified.[38] Though studies such as the Tuskegee syphilis experiment, done on unknowing individuals who were withheld curative treatment, indeed reveal some physicians to have dubious motives in their interactions with patients, a cartoonish image of physician as villain came to have a life of its own in illness narratives. Storylines portraying the doctor as an unscrupulous villain and the patient as virtuous hero became common.[39]

Patients were not the only ones dissatisfied with the biological reductionism of medical care. Clinicians such as Eric Cassell, Edward Pellegrino, Arthur Frank, and Rita Charon also expressed displeasure with the impersonal biomedical model. Rather than taking a positivist approach to medicine, these physicians highlight the value of care and healing in addition to the value of cure and treatment of disease. Dr. Cassell focuses on healing as the central concern of medicine, but he notes that even well-meaning clinicians who want to be patient centered do not know what this means or how to do it. The goal of care is ultimately the well-being of the patient. Yet well-being cannot be reduced to mere QOL (quality-of-life) measures.[40] For Cassell, well-being involves being able to live your authentic life rather than being only disease-free. He writes, "Well-being is related to feelings of being oneself (with oneself and in relation to others), being able to live life as desired, and feeling able to accomplish what is considered important."[41] While such care is commendable, the question of whether or not it is appropriate to expect physicians to assist us in pursuing our good life remains. For Cassell, the answer is plain: The doctor's role is humanistic and involves both cure of disease and the relief of suffering. For Charon, literature is the medium for developing empathy and awareness of the interiority of patients for clinicians, leading to the kind of care Cassell promotes.

CLINICIANS AND THE PRACTICE OF NARRATIVE MEDICINE

Narrative medicine involves the study of different modalities of written texts, including literature, poetry, and dramatic works, with the overarching goal of understanding patients and their experience of the clinical encounter. According to Rita Charon, physician and literature scholar who coined the term, narrative medicine "provides health care professionals with practical wisdom in comprehending what patients endure in illness and what they themselves undergo in the care of the sick."[42] The underlying premise is that the study of literature will improve one's ability to provide care by developing one's listening skills and skills of clinical attention. Through reading literature one can become a better listener and a more attentive clinician, giving attention to the role of understanding, reciprocity, and connection in the clinical encounter. With special attention given to the work of Henry James, who calls the act of listening a practice in being an "empty cup of attention," Charon maintains that learning to be a close reader of texts can offer a way to develop one's clinical skills. Because reading fiction involves considering events from multiple perspectives, Charon maintains that developing narrative competence can cultivate a person's sense of empathy.[43] Dwelling in a theoretical, fictitious dimension and encountering the inner experience of characters can expand a clinician's awareness of the inner experience of patients and family members. As Tod Chambers notes in *The Fiction of Bioethics* there is no binary between theory and practice in narrative medicine.[44] For clinicians, practice is informed by theory, and theory is applied to care and models of education. The practice according to Charon is the "reading, writing, telling, and receiving of stories."[45] The conceptual framework behind this practice relies on an understanding of the person as a narrative being, an understanding of selfhood that I examine in this chapter.

For patients, narrative medicine can offer a vehicle to reflect on and share one's experience with illness and medical treatment. The rise of autobiographical patient narratives in the United States occurred largely in response to how patients were viewed and treated by their medical caregivers. Some patients felt neglected and unheard, and they believe this experience had an effect on their well-being. After examining the history of medical pedagogy in the United States, it is apparent that physicians were providing, and continue to provide, what they were trained to believe was medically appropriate clinical care at the time. Today, however, views on what promotes patient care have expanded to include an approach to patient identity that values more than just the body and a disease-model of medicine.

CLINICAL PEDAGOGY IN NARRATIVE MEDICINE

Narrative methods in medicine are based on the following claims: one, that empathic presence can be cultivated and, two, that the imagination is a valid source of moral understanding and not one to be discarded as subjective, relative, and nonrational, as Mark Johnson claims so well in his text defending the place of the moral imagination in ethics.[46] Johnson and Ricoeur share the view that one can dwell within a story and approach literature as a source for ethical reflection. Similarly, literature can be used as a source for clinical reflection. Johnson notes, "Narrative is not just an explanatory device, but it is actually constitutive of the way we experience things. No moral theory can be adequate if it does not take into account the narrative character of our experience."[47] Using narrative methods in the clinical encounter calls for three primary steps: recognizing the human being as a narrative being, learning to be a close reader (of texts and human communication), and learning to invite the patient's story and engage in the work of interpretation along with the patient.

The goals of narrative medicine include cultivating the ability to demonstrate empathic presence with patients and deepening one's ability to listen to patients such that one can listen for what is being said beneath the words and to notice what remains unsaid. Ricoeur's words on the pedagogical function of narrative are easily applied to the clinical context. He looks to Aristotle's

Poetics, noting that Aristotle "did not hesitate to say that every well-told story teaches something; even more, he said that stories reveal universal aspects of the human condition."[48] Though for Aristotle the form of knowledge offered through *poesis* is considered as a lesser form of knowledge than that provided by logic, it is nevertheless knowledge, as Ricoeur emphasizes.[49] Ricoeur describes narrative intelligence as a type of "phronetic intelligence" distinct from theoretical intelligence, making it particularly useful for clinicians doing the on-the-ground work of patient care.[50]

Using narrative methods in clinical education, through the use of literature or learning to view the clinician/patient counter as one that is narratively based, can develop empathic awareness for clinicians, specifically the ability to recognize the separate, inner world of the patient. Scholars in narrative medicine celebrate the work of novelist Henry James because he was able to describe with nuance the distinct, though ambiguous and often inwardly held, points of view of his characters.[51] His work highlights the variety of interpretations that can exist within characters or readers. He describes the ways interpretations can vary in his preface to *Portrait of a Lady*:

> The house of fiction has in short not one window, but a million. . . . [A]t each of them stands a figure with a pair of eyes, or at least with a field-glass, . . . insuring to the person making use of it an impression distinct from every other. He and his neighbors are watching the same show, but one seeing more where the other sees less, one seeing black where the other sees white, one seeing big where the other sees small, one seeing coarse where the other sees fine.[52]

A narrative pedagogy can point to the existence of, as well as the limits to subjectivity for the physician, recognizing that one's diagnosis might be one possible interpretation among others can be an awareness cultivated through the use of narrative-based clinical training. In *The Fragility of Goodness*, Martha Nussbaum speaks about this possibility when she looks to using literature as a source for moral understanding. Literature can teach the reader/clinician to consider ethical quandaries or concerns from different perspectives, moving beyond one's own limited understanding. In her interpretation of *Antigone*, Nussbaum looks to what the chorus reminds us when they, considering the ethical crisis that Antigone and Creon are involved in, say, "Looking at this strange portent, I think on both sides." For Nussbaum, a perspective that can hold fragments within it, that can take on and embody different viewpoints, holds value when it comes to deliberating well:

> The image of learning expressed in this style, like the picture of reading required by it, stresses responsiveness and an attention to complexity; it discourages the search for the simple and, above all, for the reductive. It suggests to us that the

world of practical choice, like the text, is articulated but never exhausted by reading; that reading must reflect and not obscure this fact that correct choice (or: good interpretation) is, first and foremost, a matter of keenness and flexibility of perception, rather than of conformity to a set of simplifying principles.[53]

Because clinicians will be interpreting a patient's story from a medical perspective with the patient, the clinician's ability to acknowledge the patient's experience and interpretation as valid is one that can be developed using narrative methods in clinical education.

Wayne Booth offers suggestions for how medical practitioners can incorporate narrative methods into the care they provide. Booth recommends that practitioners, in addition to their diagnostic work (or as part of their diagnostic work), attend to the stories their patients tell and that practitioners should be aware of how they are perceived by patients. He also encourages practitioners to look to literature as a way of flexing their empathic awareness and as a means by which one can increase self-awareness as a care-provider.[54] Julia Connelly similarly speaks about how a clinician can gain narrative knowledge:

> The physician must also struggle for a deep awareness and understanding of herself, both her personality and her true self. Here physicians need the capacity for being present with the patient, an understanding of their own personal intentions, beliefs, and values and the ability to set them aside in order to focus on the patient, the commitment to care for the patient as a person, and an acceptance of feelings as an integral aspect of patient care. . . . To engage in practice designed to enhance self-knowledge is a commitment to improve health care. Without narrative, deep human contact is very difficult, especially in the setting of present-day medical practice.[55]

Charon uses the language of narrative competence to describe the ability to hear, interpret, and act on the story of another, and she maintains that this competence can be taught to clinicians.[56] She views narrative competence as the ability to "recognize, absorb, interpret, and be moved by the stories of illness."[57] Use of narrative method provides a way for the clinician to practice the imaginative, empathic turn toward another through actively receptive listening.[58] By being heard a patient can feel recognized by the clinician. Hilde Lindemann Nelson makes a similar claim about the power of recognition that can occur through narrative, suggesting that many individuals, particularly women, feel invisible because their lives are named for them by those speaking on their behalf.[59] By giving an individual patient an opportunity to offer his or her own narrative, the clinician creates a space for recognition of the patient's individual value.

Ricoeur's understanding of the tasks involved in the hermeneutical approach to literature does not have to be an approach limited to written documents. His recommendations for engaging with literature can be applied to those who are engaging with patients. He says, "A literary hermeneutics worth of the name must assume a threefold task . . . of understanding . . . explanation . . . and application. In contrast to a superficial view, reading must not be confined to the field of application even if this field does reveal the end of the hermeneutical process; instead reading must pass through all three stages."[60] Similarly, a physician engages in a hermeneutical process of understanding, explanation, and application when the physician attempts to interpret the patient's medical concerns, explain what is happening medically, and then applying a plan of care. The dynamic is one based on interpretation of the patient's needs and what will be therapeutic for the patient.[61]

THE NARRATIVE SELF FOR RICOEUR

The narrative self functions through what Ricoeur, expanding on Aristotle's concept of *mythos*, calls emplotment. In his essay "Life: A Story in Search of a Narrator," Ricoeur defines what he means when he describes the dimensions of plot and plotting as being central to the narrative structure of selfhood. It is, he emphasizes, an operative process, not a fixed one. It is also an integrative process. The process of plotting has three movements: first, it involves a synthesis of various incidents within a unitive narrative arc; second, it involves the synthetic processing of both the concordant and the discordant (the discordant being that which is unexpected); third, it involves integrating events into a timeline.[62] He sums up the act of plotting as follows: "From this analysis of a story as a synthesis of the dissimilar, then, we may retain three traits: the mediation between multiple incidents and the singular story accomplished in the plot; the primacy of concord over discord; finally, the struggle between succession and configuration."[63] Ricoeur, in *Time and Narrative* 3, uses the language of mimesis—mimesis as prefiguration, configuration and refiguration—to describe emplotment.

Ricoeur's words on emplotment are germane for clinicians because clinicians are encountering patients whose lives have been disrupted by illness; they are engaged in the dynamic process of negotiating discordant elements of their lives (breakdown of the external self, which cannot be neatly separated from the internal self, via illness or accident) into their narrative. They can experience the loss of possibilities for one's future self, and the anticipated loss of time.[64] Ricoeur's words about adjusting our expectations regarding how our lives will unfold speak directly to the experience of those struggling with physical and mental impairment who have to reshape their stories. He writes, "One gains understanding of such composition (of discord and concord) through the act of following the story; to follow a story is a very complex business, unceasingly guided by expectations concerning its course, expectations that we gradually adjust in line with the unfolding of the story right up until it reaches its conclusion."[65] For Ricoeur, the thought behind this negotiation of the disruptions and upheavals of one's life into a coherent story is the idea of the self striving for a narrative unity or wholeness.[66]

Though Ricoeur describes human beings as reflexive, self-narrating beings, he maintains that we are not authors of our own life-narratives.[67] Lisa Jones disagrees with Ricoeur on this point, noting that, although it is true that humans do not have narrative control or awareness of the events of birth and death, there is room to claim that humans can be understood as the authors of their own narratives, particularly in the activity of planning for the future. She terms this act, *figuration*, following and supplementing Ricoeur's language of the threefold nature of mimesis as prefiguration, configuration, and refiguration.[68] For Ricoeur, we can be narrators of our lives, but not authors. For Jones, we can be *both* narrators and authors, our authorship coming from our plotting for the future and bringing this future into being.[69] Jones offers a considerable sense of human agency here—not all have the luxury of hope in the future or the potential of being, in Jones's words, "hero" of their own story.[70] Also, Ricoeur does speak of the human beings as yearning, "intending," forward-reaching beings in *Fallible Man*, though his interest in the goal-oriented human is more on the *limits* of the ability to reach these goals, primarily the limit of finitude.[71] He sees the human as somewhat more vulnerable than Jones does, the finite, beheld body being the primary signifier of this vulnerability.[72, 73]

In addition to viewing the structure of the self as one shaped by narrativity, Ricoeur names the self as a *suffering* self, expanding beyond the idea of the cogito as being central to selfhood.[74] There is one element of his philosophy of selfhood, however, that may differ from that posited in bioethics, bioethics *qua* principlism, and this is his view of agency as both active and passive. Principlism, with its emphasis on autonomy, relies on the active form of agency but can overlook the other dimension of the human person—our passivity. Passivity can be understood in a variety of ways that are both external, such as being born into a structure that preceded us (language and finitude are central for Ricoeur here) and our being subject to experiences in life that befall us, a terminal diagnosis, for instance. Passivity can also be understood as a form of agency, and this is how Ricoeur approaches the self's passivity. Passive agency is a relational mode of being. Ricoeur lifts up the receptive capacity of the self: one receives the attestation of another.[75] He also uses the language of testimony as that which is given and received—one's moral personhood coming from both giving an address and receiving the address of another.[76]

Ricouer's work connects with those doing narrative ethics in medicine in that he is interested in both structures of selfhood and in practical experience and ethical modes of being in the world. Ricoeur speaks directly to the clinician/patient encounter in his piece, "Prudential Judgment, Deontological Judgment and Reflexive Judgment in Medical Ethics."[77] In this essay, Ricoeur talks about the dyadic relationship between the physician and patient, a relationship that, though it is not a symmetrical relationship, can be seen as a form of covenant. Intentional about word-choice, Ricoeur uses the language of prudential here (*prudentia* as the Latin form of the Greek *phronesis*) and he also uses the language of pact to describe the patient/clinician relationship:

> What, we will ask, is the ethical core of this singular encounter? It is the pact of confidentiality that joins together this patient and this doctor. At this prudential level, we will not yet speak of contracts and medical secrets but of a *pact of care based on trust*. Now this pact seals an original process. At the start a gap and even a remarkable dissymmetry separate the two protagonists: on one side, the one who knows and knows what to do; on the other, the one who is suffering.[78]

For Ricoeur, a bridge exists between the two subjects, and this bridge is the pact between them. The pact is based on trust and promise, the latter being an idea central to Ricoeur's understanding of the self as presented in *Oneself as Another*. The patient promises to respect the judgment of the physician and the prescribed plan of care, and the physician promises to offer the best treatment available to the patient.[79] Both are united in common cause against the illness and because of this alliance there is reason to trust the other. Ricoeur, not being a purist, recognizes that this relationship is fragile and can be threatened by mistrust on either side. This is why he calls for the "co-responsibility of the partners in the pact."[80] Of note, in *Time and Narrative* Ricoeur also calls for trust in the act of refiguration that occurs when one reads a text, trusting to follow where the text leads as a reliable source, even if one will ultimately reject the text's truth claims.[81]

In addition to his thoughts on trust and promise, Ricoeur's understanding of mimesis also holds value for narrative method in medicine, particularly his understanding of mimesis,[3] where the intersection of the world of the text and the world of the reader occurs. David Hall summarizes Ricoeur's thoughts on what can occur when reading a narrative. Reading a narrative is "to imaginatively inhabit the world that is presented by the text. More importantly, to read is to be taught by the text, to allow one's practical understanding to be guided by the narrative's horizon of experience."[82] The third mimetic move captures what ideally can occur when the clinician engages empathically with the patient, when, within the clinical encounter the clinician can imaginatively consider the perspective and experience of the patient. The clinician cannot fully know or have the patient's experience, yet there can nevertheless be movement toward understanding the patient's concerns from a place of deep listening, curiosity, and compassion.

Though a clinician can make the empathic step to understanding the world of his or her patient, this does not mean that the clinician has full access or can know with certainty what the patient experiences. Just as literature and sacred texts cannot be fully comprehended, offering boundless material for reflection and interpretation, the inner world of others cannot be fully known. Naming the plurality of interpretation that exists in literature can be a way of understanding the diversity of human experience that exists when one encounters another person. Ricoeur's concept of narrative identity and the process of emplotment can serve as a resource for examining models of patient identity in narrative medicine. A clinician's awareness of both the limits of one's own understanding and the existence of the separate world of the other can be developed through the use of literature in clinical education and through learning to view one's relationship with a patient as an interpretive encounter.

MEDICAL ETHICS AND CLINICAL PRACTICE

Principlism as a modality of decision-making in medical ethics formally began with the publication of Tom Beauchamp and John Childress' *Principles of Biomedical Ethics* in 1979.[83] In brief, principlism centers on four concepts: autonomy, beneficence, nonmaleficence, and justice. While principlism undoubtedly did a great deal of good in creating a platform for patient's rights, particularly through the establishment of informed consent, the method can be seen as a minimalist approach to the complex dynamics that occur between patients and clinicians.[84] Principlism has also been critiqued as offering something of an ethical checklist for clinicians creating a scenario in which, once the four categories have been considered, other ethical issues are not taken into account, such as when two of the principles might conflict.[85] The principles can be critiqued for being too neat and limited, as well as, on the other end of the spectrum, for being too general and open.[86] Recognizing the limits of principlism does not mean that the model should be jettisoned entirely. However, the model can be improved by a more nuanced understanding of, to use Paul Ramsey's term, the patient as person.[87]

Many clinicians recognize the limits of principlism in terms of how much the framework can provide for informing the diagnostic encounter. The term "narrative ethics" is also used in various ways. Literary scholars like Wayne Booth use the term "narrative ethics" to describe how one can critically approach texts and use them as sources for ethical understanding and evaluation, recognizing that a reader can make claims about the ethical function of texts.[88] Martha Nussbaum looks to literature as a narrative source for moral understanding. Other scholars such as Hilde Lindemann Nelson, Arthur Frank, Howard Brody, and Rita Charon uphold the idea of the patient as a person whose being in the world is marked by narration. Their claims often have an implicit or explicit ethical appraisal of the medical model.

The narrative understanding of the self asserted by Paul Ricoeur, particularly in *Oneself as Another* and in the third volume of *Time and Narrative*, can supplement medical ethics, but can also inform how patients are understood and treated in the medical model of care.[89] While principlism highlights the autonomous mode of being of a person, Ricoeur, while not negating this view, turns his attention to the narrative practices individuals engage in. A person engages in taking the fragments of one's life and attempting to unify them into a coherent whole—though this unity is never fully achieved as an individual continually engages in the process of reinterpreting the past, present, and future. One can imagine how a patient might engage in this narrative process after receiving a life-changing diagnosis that disrupts the narrative the person envisioned for his or her future. These two concepts, narrativity and autonomy, are not in opposition, and the respect for autonomy is crucial to medical ethics. However, the language of autonomy does not take into account the rupture that can occur when one experiences physical or mental illness, or the loss of autonomy that might concurrently be experienced with an illness, the need of an ALS person to receive care as a dependent, for instance. Ricoeur's view of the centrality of hermeneutics supplements, but does not replace, the centrality of autonomy in the medical model. Ricoeur notes that narratives, while they can order lives in accordance with moral norms, cannot "by themselves *found* ethics."[90] Through narrativity Ricoeur does not offer a replacement for principalist ethics; rather, he offers a way to include, but expand beyond, the category of autonomy as the salient feature of a patient's being.

Scholars in narrative medicine present a critique of medical pedagogy and practice and in so doing provide resources for ethical analysis. Behind normative claims that the practice of medicine can be improved by mindfully attending to a patient's narrative hides the claim that medicine offers an inadequate approach to patient care. When advocates of narrative medicine claim that reading literature nurtures empathic regard for patients, what then does this claim suggest about clinicians that have a science-based focus? Narrative approaches to identity formation and clinical practice create space for uncertainty; therefore, easy binaries between the virtuous scholar-physicians and the heartless scientist-physicians call for nuance. A contribution of a narrative-based approach is that it offers resources for engaging with the gaps and gray areas in medical knowledge and in medical ethics. Drawing on an approach that allows for multivalent understandings of personhood, one can claim that there is no pure approach to clinical care, either on the side of empathic clinicians or on the side of those who prefer a posture of clinical detachment.

A view of the narrative self can serve as a reminder to take into account the complexity of a person's situation, one that may not have a solution or even a diagnosis. While there is a desire in medicine to have certainty, a desire made manifest though, for instance, over-testing patients, a narrative, hermeneutically centered approach to the relationship between clinician and patient functions with the awareness that absolute certainty is not always possible when making a diagnosis or trying to understand the suffering of a patient. An understanding of the narrative self and the narrative encounter recognizes that in the diagnostic encounter and particularly in ethical dilemmas, there is not necessarily one "right" diagnosis or one "right" answer. There can be multiple entry points into understanding a patient's experience. Laurie Zoloth points to the value of sacred texts as a reminder that ambiguity, not certainty, is what marks human experience. "Biblical texts," she says, "with their unsettled questions and the dark lacunae and the flawed heroes are a template for the lacunae of medicine and allow for a midrashic, interpretive and contextual analysis of the medical narratives that we are called on to reflect upon."[91]

Taking into account the particularity of an individual's story involves time and close attention. Being attentive to a patient's story can take more time than a physical exam. However, listening to the patient's concerns may save time by decreasing over-testing and it also may reveal other medical concerns, such as psychosocial and spiritual concerns, that warrant treatment or referral to chaplains or mental health providers. Also, to continue the conversation about medical ethics, narrativity brings a human component to the rights-based structure of principlism. A narrative approach is not meant to replace principlism, only to supplement the model. If anything, narrativity highlights the agency of a patient and falls under the principle of autonomy.

Tod Chambers names two distinct approaches to narrative medical ethics, and, though the two are often conflated, they have different goals and methods.[92] One, developed by Kathryn Montgomery, situates itself as taking a distanced, more observational view of narrative medicine. Descriptive in approach, Montgomery's style offers a philosophy of medicine rather than an ethical analysis of how medicine ought to be performed. Rita Charon presents another approach, one based on practice rather than observation. Charon's work, particularly her books *Stories Matter* and *Narrative Medicine*, is a confluence of literary theory, clinical application, medical pedagogy, and medical ethics.[93, 94] Offering an ethical analysis of how medicine could be improved, she calls on the clinician to develop narrative competence. Her interest is in how the clinical encounter can be improved through the use of literature. Specifically, her focus is on the use of literature in the education of clinicians. Charon's work falls into the domain of ethics, particularly virtue ethics, in the sense that she believes increasing narrative training in medicine will develop a clinician's sense of "humility, accountability, [and] empathy."[95] Through reading groups, narrating one's experience with patients, and the use of narrative curriculum in medical training students learn to be close readers of text.[96] Anne Hudson Jones describes the questions that a narrative curriculum can teach medical students to ask:

> Who is the narrator? Is the narrator reliable? From what perspective or point of view is the story told? What does this perspective leave out? Who are the other potential narrators of this story? What might their perspectives add? How can differences between narrators' stories be reconciled? What do individual readers bring to the story that influences their interpretations? How can differing interpretations be reconciled? If they cannot be reconciled, how should a reader handle such ambiguity? What patterns emerge from the accumulating details, repetitions, images, and metaphors? That is, how does a skilled reader learn to recognize significant details that cohere in a pattern of meaning that makes sense of the whole?[97]

Assumed in this approach to education is the correlation between attending closely to texts and attending closely to patients. Charon recommends parallel charting for clinicians, in which a medical history is expanded to include extra-clinical observations.[98] A benefit of this approach is that those teaching in medical schools can then see how students are interpreting their patient's behavior, possibly overreaching in their interpretations, and the educator can then "diagnose" concerns having to do with the clinician's training.

According to scholars in the field, one of the benefits of clinical training in narrative method is that it will nurture an empathic response in a clinician. The premise underlying this view is that by learning to understand the world from a fictional character's or narrator's perspective, the clinician will be able to understand the patient's perspective of illness. As Rita Charon says, "to know what patients endure at the hands of illness and therefore to be of clinical help requires that doctors *enter* the worlds of their patients, if only imaginatively, and to see and interpret these worlds from the patients' point of view."[99] She is working to mitigate the clinical detachment that can result from scientistic medical training by working with physicians to take into account multiple points of view.

Charon recognizes that narrative competence is a sophisticated skill that requires some self-awareness.[100] One has to have the desire to develop one's ability to listen and communicate. In ways, though, this is a reverse catch-22. The desire points to the reality that the clinician already has an awareness of the experience of the other. However, not all individuals have such awareness. "Alexithymia" is the term Howard Spiro gives to clinicians who are out of touch with their own emotions in addition to being detached or unaware of the emotional states of their patients.[101]

In a clinical encounter centered on narrativity, the narrative self manifests through dialogue with a clinician. Charon speaks about the intimacy that can exist in these encounters. Though honorable, some questions about narrative medicine call for consideration. Can a patient be fully known by a clinician? How does the asymmetry of power come into play? In what ways does narrative medicine inflate the role of the clinician and violate a vulnerable patient's inner sanctum? The limited nature of relationality is also recognized by figures such as Judith Butler and Levinas, using the language of "otherness." Some, Eric Cassell, notably, believe this emphasis on distance, opacity, and otherness is overstated. Cassell believes patients can be known and that physicians can make excuses for their lack of engagement by emphasizing the unknowability of patients.[102]

Charon recognizes that physicians cannot have the final say when it comes to understanding a patient's narrative—that there is a gap between the clinician and patient and that there is then a need to corroborate their interpretation of patient's experience. She says, "I have come slowly to appreciate that patients should be the curators of what we write about them." Thus she gives them a copy of her note and asks them to consider what she has written.[103] One can ask, though, is there even a need for empathy in the clinical encounter or is it nice but unnecessary, even intrusive? Some claim that it is ultimately not the role of a physician to provide emotional or metaphysical support and that not all patients are interested in their physician being present in this way. As Ronald Andiman notes in "Midrash and Medicine,"

> Patients have their own expectations of a doctor, and many patients would actually be impatient with an extended process of communication; they value efficiency over breadth or depth, especially if they don't think of their problem as complex. Some patients, because of a heavily defended psyche or because of their value system, merely want to get a brief "answer"; they get their emotional support elsewhere or perhaps not at all. The point is, one size (of verbal discourse) doesn't fit all.[104]

The important thing to note about narrative medicine is that not all patients are interested in a dialogical encounter with clinicians. If we pull back from seeing the detachment of clinicians as a problem, we can ask whether a meaning-based response is necessary for the clinical encounter. Though the ability to listen and communicate well is a skill and can be, and in many cases is, taught in medical school, empathic presence that has a spiritual, emotional, or meaning-based value, is not what all patients prefer.

Physicians may not be trained or have the time available to listen to patients' narratives and to interpret them beyond the medical, yet there is nevertheless value in narrative training in that it teaches physicians to take into account information that falls outside the narrow domain of biological positivism. As Eric Cassell recognizes, physicians work with more than just medical facts; they also work with meaning and questions of morality. Larry Miller likens the work of medicine to the deductive reasoning of Sherlock Holmes, a type of speculative reasoning that creates a narrative out of disparate, but possibly related, pieces of evidence. Though a meaning-based response is ultimately not necessary for the clinical encounter to be successful (for diagnosis and treatment to occur), this dynamic can still be what the patient desires. Like attentive dialogue, touch can also be considered superfluous to the medical encounter, but it is nevertheless significant for patients and calls for taking into account.[105]

One of the values of using narrativity in clinical reasoning is there is recognition that a patient's life existed before the clinical encounter or medical event occurred and that it will continue to affect the patient's life afterward. A narrative understanding of care sees the medical moment as one moment in a patient's life. The concept of narrativity is particularly valuable for clinicians because it takes into account how selfhood is shaped in relation to time.[106] For some, time can be understood chronologically in a linear fashion, but others recognize that we move back and forth in time in terms of how we construct our understanding of self. Ricoeur, for instance, uses the language of mimesis—a process involving prefiguration, configuration, and refiguration—to build on and nuance the Aristotelian notion that we are agents in our own lives.[107] Time is understood in a linear way, but it is also understood as at the same time containing past, present, and future constructions of the self. That is, one can think of whom one *desires* to be. For Ricoeur, there is both the fixed, concrete self, located in linear time, and the fluid, imagined self, that exists, in ways, as a fiction.

Some scholars in narrative medicine understand time in terms of phases of life. Arthur Frank notes that illness narratives can be interpreted in terms of restitution, quest, dealing with chaos.[108] He identifies the postmodern self as the self that tells one's own story.[109] Kathlyn Conway describes some illness narratives as "narratives of triumph"—she recognizes a pattern in illness narratives and she finds this formula problematic because it can easily become prescriptive.[110] The "narratives of triumph" involve a patient experiencing what could be called a fall and redemption (though Conway uses secular language). The patient is well and in standard health, then experiences the rupture and shock of a diagnosis, then copes and conquers the process. Restoration and healing have been achieved.[111] She links her term "narratives of triumph" to Arthur Frank's term "restitution narratives," stories that share the same predictable pattern: "Yesterday I was healthy, today I'm sick, but tomorrow I'll be healthy again."[112] Ultimately, this pattern does not hold for all patients, though, particularly chronically ill and terminal patients. This does not mean that restoration, healing, and hope cannot be redefined in a new way however. For some patients, their hope for a cure may transition to hope for intentional time spent with family or a visit to a beloved park. The hope is still there, but the goal is no longer oriented to the body, but oriented to meaning. Again, the sense of self and agency assumed by both Conway and Frank is not available to all patients.

CONCLUSION

Western medicine is deeply teleological, a quest-based model structured on a linear process that includes diagnosis, treatment, and ultimately, cure. Patients, though, do not necessarily have a goal-based vision of care, or their goals may not be diagnosis and acute treatment, but understanding and guidance about how to live with an illness when curative care does not exist as a possibility. This is particularly true for chronically ill or terminal patients who do not fit into a goal-based paradigm. Patients turned to narrative-based responses to their experience of impersonal clinical care. Some schools of thought in the medical humanities look to the patient as a more authentic or valid source of medical information, one that is closer to the truth than the accounts provided by clinicians. Patient narratives can also serve a therapeutic or social function for the patient, providing a means of taking back one's authority or a means of connecting a patient to others who have shared their experience of feeling dehumanized. As a source of ethical reflection, patient narratives can point to the need for systemic change in the medical system, offering a normative critique of care in the form of a personal testimony. Patient accounts can also be sources of ethical self-evaluation, as I explore in the chapter on life review in hospice. While many patients and clinicians find value in the narrative features of health care, there are patients who are cognitively unable to offer any sort of understandable narrative or account at all, and it is this group of patients that I address in chapter 4.

In following chapters, I continue to examine narrative-based concepts of patient identity and practice and the value of narrative medicine for clinicians.

I focus on the process of life review in hospice, and then turn to the limits of narrative practices for patients who are unable or limited in their abilities to engage in the process. Additionally, I explore the religious dimension of patients as one that calls for recognition in the study of narrative medicine. When trying to make sense of the world around us, particularly in times of unexpected distress, we look to reasons why our bodies and minds are not working the way we would like them to. Some of the reasons are medical, but many are religious, a reason why chaplains are included in medical care teams in hospitals and hospice care. There are also deeply valuable sources of religious literature, such as the Psalms, that create space in narrative medicine for the recognition of darkness and ambiguity in the lives of both patients and clinicians.

NOTES

1. Abraham Flexner and Daniel Berkeley Updike, *Medical Education in the United States and Canada: A Report to the Carnegie Foundation for the Advancement of Teaching* (New York City: Merrymount Press, 1910).

2. Thomas Patrick Duffy, "The Flexner Report—100 Years Later," *The Yale Journal of Biology and Medicine* 84, no. 3 (2011): 269.

3. Theodor Billroth, Leon Banov, and Kellogg Speed, *The Medical Sciences in the German Universities: A Study in the History of Civilization* (New York: The Macmillan Company, 1924). Duffy notes that this text was central to Flexner's understanding of the German model of medical education.

4. Milton James Lewis, *Medicine and Care of the Dying: A Modern History* (Oxford; New York: Oxford University Press, 2007), 46–47

5. The term "evidence-based medicine" (EBM) was first used by David M. Eddy in a 1990 article in the *Journal of the American Medical Association*. The turn toward evidence-based medicine began earlier than this, however, and Flexner and Fishbein's views of medicine align with those later asserted in EBM. David M. Eddy, "Practice Policies: Guidelines for Methods," *JAMA* 263, no. 13 (1990): 1839–41.

6. Eric J. Cassell, *The Nature of Healing: The Modern Practice of Medicine* (Oxford; New York: Oxford University Press, 2013), 83. I use the theological language of Donatistism to point to the Augustinian idea that the personal failings of the priest are irrelevant to the nature of sacrament; the priest functions in a technical role where his personality does not come into play. Physicians can be seen similarly in a technical role as scientists.

7. Eric J. Cassell, *The Nature of Suffering and the Goals of Medicine* (New York: Oxford University Press, 1991), x.

8. Morris Fishbein, *Medical Follies: An Analysis of the Foibles of Some Healing Cults, Including Osteopathy, Homeopathy, Chiropractic, and the Electronic Reactions of Abrams, with Essays on the Anti-Vivisectionists, Health Legislation, Physical Culture, Birth Control, and Rejuvenation* (New York: Boni & Liveright, 1925). For

how his work applies to more current trends, see his text *The New Medical Follies: An Encyclopedia of Cultism and Quackery in These United States, with Essays on the Cult of Beauty, the Craze for Reduction, Rejuvenation, Eclecticism, Bread and Dietary Fads, Physical Therapy, and a Forecast as to the Physician of the Future* (New York: Boni & Liveright, 1927; New York: AMS Press, 1977).

9. Milton James Lewis, *Medicine and the Care of the Dying: A Modern History* (Oxford: Oxford Univ. Press, 2007), 34.

10. Lewis, *Medicine and the Care of the Dying*, 33.

11. Ibid., 34.

12. Institute for Professionalism Inquiry Conference Proceedings et al., *Toward Healing: Virtuous Practice, Spiritual Care and Narrative Medicine* (Akron, OH: Institute for Professionalism Inquiry, 2005), 6–22.

13. To describe the toll on clinicians that comes with repeatedly responding to complex medical needs, the term "compassion fatigue" was coined by Carla Joinson in a 1992 article, "Coping with Compassion Fatigue," *Nursing* 22, no. 4, 118–20. The term was broadened to include other caregivers, such as those in behavioral medicine, or informal caregivers providing emotional labor by C. R. Figley in *Compassion Fatigue: Coping with Secondary Traumatic Stress Disorder in Those Who Treat the Traumatized* (New York, NY: Brunner Mazel, 1995). Compassion fatigue continues to play a role in clinician and caregiver burnout. See T. Shanafelt, "Enhancing Meaning in Work: A Prescription for Preventing Physician Burnout and Promoting Patient-Centered Care," *JAMA* 302 (2009): 1338–40. For a review of the literature on compassion fatigue, see N. Najjar, L. W. Davis, K. Beck-Coon, and C. C. Doebbeling, "Compassion Fatigue: A Review of the Research to Date and Relevance to Cancer-care Providers," *Journal of Health Psychology* 14 (2009): 267–77.

14. Jack Coulehan, "From Virtue to Narrative: The Art of Healing," in *Toward Healing: Virtuous Practice, Spiritual Care and Narrative Medicine* (Akron, OH: Institute for Professionalism Inquiry, 2005), 9.

15. Coulehan, "From Virtue to Narrative: The Art of Healing," 11

16. Ibid., 11.

17. Ibid., 15.

18. Rita Charon, "Narrative Medicine: A Model for Empathy, Reflection, Profession, and Trust," *JAMA* 286 (2001): 1897–1902. See also Charon's forward in *Narrative in Health Care: Healing Patients, Practitioners, and Profession, and Community* (Oxford: Radcliffe Publishing, 2008), ix–xii. For more on the cultivation of empathy for clinicians, see the following by Sayantani DasGupta and Rita Charon, "Personal Illness Narratives: Using Reflective Writing to Teach Empathy," *Academic Medicine* 79 (2004): 351–56.

19. Sayantani DasGupta and Marsha Hurst, *Stories of Illness and Healing: Women Write Their Bodies* (Kent, OH: Kent State University Press, 2007), 212. Additionally, Christina Puchalski writes extensively on the need to teach clinicians about the extra-medical needs of patients, particularly spiritual and religious needs. See the following articles: Christina Puchalski, "Spirituality and Medicine: Curricula in Medical Education," *Journal of Cancer Education: The Official Journal of the American Association for Cancer Education*, 21, no. 1 (2006): 14–18; Christina Puchalski and D. Larson, "Developing

Curricula in Spirituality and Medicine," *Academic Medicine: Journal of the Association of American Medical Colleges* 73, no. 9 (1998): 970–74; and, S. Levin, D. Larson, and C. Puchalski, "Religion and Spirituality in Medicine: Research and Education," *JAMA : The Journal of the American Medical Association* 278, no. 9 (1997): 792–93.

20. Ann Jurecic, *Illness as Narrative* (Pittsburgh: University of Pittsburgh Press, 2012), 1.

21. Jurecic, *Illness as Narrative*, 18–19.

22. Following standards set in place following the publication of the Flexner report.

23. Richard Zaner, "Medicine and Dialogue," *The Journal of Medicine and Philosophy* 15, no. 3 (1990): 303. Zaner critiques the medical materialism of "applied biology." The term originated with Donald Seldin in 1973.

24. Anne Hunsaker Hawkins, *Reconstructing Illness: Studies in Pathography* (West Lafayette, Ind.: Purdue University Press, 1993), 21–22.

25. Cassell, *The Nature of Healing: The Modern Practice of Medicine*, xii.

26. Clifford Geertz, *The Interpretation of Cultures: Selected Essays* (New York: Basic Books, 1973). The concept of a medical culture, involving the experience of both patients and clinicians in the context of health care, took form after the publication of this text.

27. Arthur Kleinman, *The Illness Narratives: Suffering, Healing, and the Human Condition* (New York: Basic Books, 1988).

28. Jerome S. Bruner, *Making Stories: Law, Literature, Life* (New York: Farrar, Straus, and Giroux, 2002), 85–86.

29. George Engel, "The Need for a New Medical Model: A Challenge for Biomedicine," *Science* 196, no. 4286 (1977): 129.

30. See Cheryl Mattingly's *Healing Dramas and Clinical Plots: The Narrative Structure of Experience* (Cambridge, UK; New York, NY: Cambridge University Press, 1998) as a resource for narrative approaches to clinician-patient relationships in occupational therapy. Byron Good and Mary Jo Delvecchio Good investigate the general practice of medicine from an anthropological perspective.

31. Alasdair MacIntyre, *After Virtue* (University of Notre Dame Press, 1981), 216.

32. MacIntyre, *After Virtue*, 204.

33. Alasdair MacIntyre, "Epistemological Crises, Dramatic Narrative, and the Philosophy of Science," *The Monist* 60, no. 4 (October 1977): 453–72; reprinted in Alasdair MacIntyre, *The Tasks of Philosophy* (Cambridge: Cambridge University Press, 2006), 3–23.

34. Paul Ricoeur, *Time and Narrative* (Chicago: University of Chicago Press, 1984), vol. 3.

35. Tom L. Beauchamp and James F. Childress, *Principles of Biomedical Ethics* (New York: Oxford University Press, 1979).

36. *The Belmont Report: Ethical Principles and Guidelines for the Protection of Human Subjects of Research*, written in 1978, established guidelines for research on human subjects, laying the groundwork for regulations established by the US Department of Health and Human Services and the establishment of Institutional Review Boards to judge the ethicality of research on human subjects. For the original Belmont Report, see

National Commission for the Protection of Human Subjects of Biomedical and Behavioral Research, Department of Health, Education and Welfare. September 30, 1978. The *Belmont Report* (Washington, DC: United States Government Printing Office).

37. Susan Reverby, *Examining Tuskegee: The Infamous Syphilis Study and its Legacy* (Chapel Hill: University of North Carolina Press, 2009), 76.

38. Paul Ramsey, *The Patient as Person: Explorations in Medical Ethics* (New Haven: Yale University Press, 1970). This ethics text was published prior to the turn to narrative in medical anthropology.

39. B. Sharf and M. Vanderford, "Illness Narratives and the Social Construction of Reality," in *Handbook of Health Communication*, ed. T. L. Thompson, A. M. Dorsey, K. I. Miller, and R. Parrott (Mahwah, NJ: Lawrence Erlbaum, 2003), 9–34.

40. The original "Quality of Life Scale" was a measure created by psychologist John Flanagan in the 1970s for the purpose of identifying levels of physical, personal, relational, and social well-being. Similar quality-of-life measures are used to manage care for those who are terminal or live with chronic illness, including chronic mental illness. For early uses of the term, see the following: John Flanagan, "Measure of Quality of Life: Current State of the Art," *Archives of Physical and Medical Rehabilitation* 63 (1982): 56–59, and Kenneth Charles Calman, "Quality of Life in Cancer Patients—An Hypothesis," *Journal of Medical Ethics* 10, no. 3 (1984): 124–27. For how the model has changed over time, see Peter Fayers and David Machin, *Quality of Life: The Assessment, Analysis and Interpretation of Patient-Reported Outcomes* (John Wiley & Sons, 2013). For how the measure is used for those with dementia, see Rebecca Ready and Brian R. Ott, "Quality of Life Measures for Dementia," *Health and Quality of Life Outcomes* 1 (2003).

41. Cassell, *The Nature of Healing: The Modern Practice of Medicine*, xiv.

42. Rita Charon, *Narrative Medicine: Honoring the Stories of Illness* (Oxford: Oxford University Press, 2008), vii.

43. Teresa Thompson, "The Applicability of Narrative Ethics," *Journal of Applied Communication Research* 37, no. 2 (May 2009): 190.

44. Chambers, *The Fiction of Bioethics*.

45. Charon, *Narrative Medicine*, vii.

46. Mark Johnson, *Moral Imagination: Implications of Cognitive Science for Ethics* (Chicago: University of Chicago Press, 1993). Johnson, following Martha Nussbaum, looks to how literature can be a vehicle for moral reflection.

47. Johnson, *Moral Imagination*, 11.

48. Ricoeur, "Life: A Story in Search of a Narrator," in *Facts and Values: Philosophical Reflections from Western and Non-Western Perspectives*, ed. M. C. Doeser and J. N. Kraay (Dordrecht: M. Nijhoff, 1986), 122–23.

49. Hille Haker in "Narrative Ethics in Health Care Chaplaincy" notes that Ricoeur is a bridge between Aristotelian poesis, in which stories are intended to represent reality, and post-modern and post-structural hermeneutics that focus on the limits of constructed stories. In *Medical Ethics in Health Care Chaplaincy: Essays*, ed. Walter Moczynski, Hille Haker, and Katrin Bentele (Berlin: Lit, 2009), 160–61.

50. Ricoeur, "Life: A Story in Search of a Narrator," 124.

51. Rita Charon, "A Momentary Watcher, or the Imperiled Reader of 'A Round of Visits,'" *Henry James Review* 29 (2008): 275–86.

52. Henry James, *The Portrait of a Lady: The Novels and Tales of Henry James* (New York: Kelley, 1970), x–xi. Quoted by Suzanne Poirier in "Voice in the Medical Narrative" in *Stories Matter*, 48–58.

53. Martha C. Nussbaum, *The Fragility of Goodness: Luck and Ethics in Greek Tragedy and Philosophy* (Cambridge: Cambridge University Press, 2001), 69.

54. Wayne Booth, "The Ethics of Medicine, as Revealed in Literature," in *Stories Matter: The Role of Narrative in Medical Ethics*, ed. Rita Charon, and Martha Montello (New York: Routledge, 2002), 18–19. Booth presents the play *W;t* by Margaret Edson, and Tolstoy's "The Death of Ivan Ilych," as texts that show the ambiguities of both patients' and clinicians' self-understanding. Regarding how to choose what literature to look to for when navigating bioethical issues, Booth recommends texts that address moral issues for both patients and clinicians rather than just advocating the stance of one side or the other.

55. Julia E. Connelly, "In the Absence of Narrative," in *Stories Matter*, 145. Connelly also speaks about the ability to hear the story of a person who has a cognitive deficit, particularly the memory lapses experienced by Alzheimer's patients. She urges the clinician to learn how to listen to what a person is attempting to communicate with their bodies, their emotional responses, and so forth without immediately moving one's attention to the patient's verbal family member, 141–42.

56. Rita Charon, "Narrative Medicine: A Model for Empathy, Reflection, Profession, and Trust," 1897–902.

57. Rita Charon, "Narrative Medicine: Attention, Representation, Affiliation," *Narrative* 13, no. 3 (2005): 262.

58. Maintaining the value of the principalist framework for medical ethics, Charon sees narrative method not as an independent method, but as a means to supplement the encounter between clinician and patient. Rita Charon, "Narrative Contributions to Medical Ethics: Recognition, Formulation, Interpretation, and Validation in the Practice of the Ethicist," in *A Matter of Principles?: Ferment in US Bioethics*, ed. Edwin DuBose, Ronald P. Hamel, and Laurence J. O'Connell (Valley Forge, PA: Trinity Press International, 1994), 260–83.

59. Hilde Lindemann Nelson, *Damaged Identities, Narrative Repair* (Ithaca, NY: Cornell University Press, 2001).

60. Ricoeur, *Time and Narrative*, vol. 3. Quoted by Mario J. Valdes in his introduction to *A Ricoeur Reader: Reflection and Imagination* (Toronto: University of Toronto Press, 1991), 21.

61. Kathryn Montgomery Hunter in *Doctor's Stories: The Narrative Structure of Medical Knowledge* (Princeton: Princeton University Press, 1991) speaks about clinician/patient relationship as an interpretive activity. See Part I in particular.

62. Ricoeur, "Life: A Story in Search of a Narrator," 122–23.

63. Ibid., 123.

64. Speaking about the loss of one's future self and the loss of one's potentiality, David Hall links to Ricoeur's idem/ipse view of the structure of the self. Hall writes

"Human existence is lived as possibility. Another way of putting this is to say that the being of the self resided in both actuality and potentiality. This then is the significance of Ricoeur's designation of the identity of the agent in terms of both sameness and selfhood. By relating these terms thought the concepts of character and self-constancy, he wove actuality and potentiality into the being of the self." In *Ricoeur and the Poetic Imperative*, 61–62.

65. Ricoeur, "Life: A Story in Search of a Narrator," 122.

66. Ricoeur, *Oneself as Another*, 143. Here he speaks of the "unity, internal structure, and completeness" as defining the activity of emplotment.

67. Ricoeur, "Life: A Story in Search of a Narrator," 131.

68. Lisa Jones, "Oneself as an Author," *Theory, Culture and Society* 27, no. 5 (2010): 49–68, 60.

69. Pointing out that prefiguration, configuration, and refiguration all work with the past, Jones notes suggests that "in order for mimesis to apply to the whole of a life (life-story), we must add the idea of *figuration*; that is, the plotting of our futures," Jones, "Oneself as an Author," 60.

70. Jones, "Oneself as an Author," 63.

71. Paul Ricoeur, *Fallible Man* (New York: Fordham University Press, 1986).

72. Ricoeur, *Fallible Man*, 19–20. I use the language of vulnerability to highlight the difference between Jones's robust view of agency and Ricoeur's tempered view. Consistent with his later works, Ricoeur, in this translation, uses the language of receptivity rather than vulnerability. He does use the language of "fragility" but Kelbley notes that he uses it to describe our existential condition as one marked by limit. See the introduction to Kelbley's translation, xxiii.

73. Rebecca Huskey's book on hope in Ricoeur's work, *Paul Ricoeur on Hope: Expecting the Good* (New York: Peter Lang, 2009) speaks about his view of the human as future-oriented with a recognition of the limits of one's future. Speaking specifically about his anthropology in *Fallible Man*, she shows how Ricoeur's perspective recognizes both our potential as agents and our limits—our strength and our fragility and, in what can be seen as a response to Jones, our capacity for "reaching intermediate goals in pursuit of an ever-retreating horizon," 59. For those with a terminal illness, hope can still be that which orients one's life, only its shape has changed. Rather than hope for accomplishment in the future, one might hope for reconciliation with family or to leave a legacy.

74. Ricoeur, *Oneself as Another*, 22. David Hall says this of the existential position Ricoeur took in his approach to the self: "Ricoeur sought to displace the question of selfhood from this quest for epistemic certainty, for positivity, that governs the debate between philosophies of *cogito* and philosophies of '*anti-cogito*.'" His language of the self as that which both acts and suffers also parallels his view of the self as both active and passive, passivity being, as Hall notes, a dimension of agency. David W. Hall, *Paul Ricoeur and the Poetic Imperative: The Creative Tension between Love and Justice* (Albany: State University of New York Press, 2007), 28–30.

75. Ricoeur, *Oneself as Another*, 339. Ricoeur names reception, discrimination, and recognition as the ethical responses called for in one's relationship to the other.

76. Paul Ricoeur and S. Lewis, *Essays on Biblical Interpretation*, ed. Mudge (Philadelphia: Fortress, 1985). See particularly chapters two and three for his understanding of testimony. Ricoeur's *From Text to Action* (Evanston, IL: Northwestern University Press, 1991) also incorporates this view of personhood.

77. Paul Ricoeur, "Prudential Judgment, Deontological Judgment and Reflexive Judgment in Medical Ethics," in *Bioethics and Biolaw, Vol. I: Judgment of Life*, ed. Peter Kemp, Jacob Rendtorff, and Niels Mattsson Johansen (Copenhagen: Rhodos, 2000).

78. Ricoeur, "Prudential Judgment," 16.

79. Ibid., 17.

80. Ibid., 18.

81. Peter Kemp, "Ethics and Narrativity," in *The Philosophy of Paul Ricoeur* ed. Lewis Edwin Hahn (Chicago: Open Court, 1995), 379–380. Kemp says, "the reader must trust the story, at least as far as a part of what it describes as truth is concerned, to the extent that he believes that life might become as the narrative describes were people to live that manner. Ricoeur stresses in general that no refiguration of the real world of acting and suffering is possible without appropriation, whether it be more or less naïve or more or less critical."

82. Hall, *Paul Ricoeur and the Poetic Imperative*, 57.

83. Beauchamp and Childress, *Principles of Biomedical Ethics*.

84. See Albert R. Jonsen's *The Birth of Bioethics* (New York: Oxford University Press, 1998) for a critique of principlism as the primary method in bioethics.

85. See P. Gardiner, "A Virtue Ethics Approach to Moral Dilemmas in Medicine," *Journal of Medical Ethics* 29, no. 5 (2003): 297–302. Gardiner expands beyond the principalist model by looking at the virtue ethics framework as one that honors the complexity of the human being and one that can offer guidance when principles conflict or are not necessarily applicable to the patient in question.

86. Martha Nussbaum in *Love's Knowledge: Essays on Philosophy and Literature* (New York: Oxford University Press, 1990) critiques modern philosophy for being overly abstract and scientifically minded, presenting "a kind of all-purpose solvent in which philosophical issues of any kind at all could be efficiently disentangled, and any conclusions neatly disengaged," 19. Her critique could also apply to principlism in bioethics and the expectation the principlism covers the gamut of bioethical issues.

87. Notably, Ramsey's text was published prior to that of Beauchamp and Childress. Ramsey in *The Patient as Person: Explorations in Medical Ethics* (New Haven, CT: Yale University Press, 1970) speaks about the need for methodological structure in bioethics and Beauchamp and Childress's now classic text can be seen as a response to Ramsey's call.

88. Booth, "The Ethics of Medicine," in *Stories Matter*, ed. Rita Charon, and Martha Montello (New York: Routledge, 2002), 10–20.

89. Paul Ricoeur, *Oneself as Another* (Chicago: University of Chicago Press, 1992) and the three-volume *Time and Narrative* (Chicago: University of Chicago Press, 1984). Ricoeur describes the different foci of the two texts: "Whereas *Time and Narrative* was mainly interested in the role of narrative in the figuration of time,

Oneself as Another is concerned with its contribution to a hermeneutics of the Self." He points particularly to the sixth study which looks to the dialectic of idem (sameness over time) and ipse (selfhood within time) as being central to his understanding of narrative identity. In Lewis Edwin Hahn's *The Philosophy of Paul Ricoeur* (Chicago: Open Court, 1995), 396–397.

90. Ricoeur, "Reply to Peter Kemp," in *The Philosophy of Paul Ricoeur* ed. Lewis Edwin Hahn (Chicago: Open Court, 1995), 397–398. He notes that norms such as the good and duty cannot be located within the narrative structure of the self, but can be added to it, facilitating a transition from narrative identity to the morally responsible self.

91. Laurie Zoloth, "Faith and Reasoning(s): Bioethics, Religion and Prophetic Necessity," in *Notes from a Narrow Ridge: Religion and Bioethics,* ed. Dena S. Davis, and Laurie Zoloth (Hagerstown, MD: University Pub. Group, 1999), 261.

92. Chambers, "Misreading Montgomery," *Atrium,* 46.

93. Rita Charon and Martha Montello, *Stories Matter: The Role of Narrative in Medical Ethics* (New York: Routledge, 2002).

94. Charon, *Narrative Medicine.*

95. Charon, *Narrative Medicine,* vii. See also Charon's "Narrative Medicine: A Model for Empathy, Reflection, Profession, and Trust," 1897–902.

96. *Stories Matter,* 161.

97. *Stories Matter,* 160–61.

98. Rita Charon, *Narrative Medicine–Honoring the Stories of Illness* (New York: Oxford University Press, 2006), 156. In parallel charting, the clinician, in addition to diagnostic charting, records the concerns of the patient in a more reflective, narrative manner. See also Rita Charon, "Narrative Medicine: Form, Function, and Ethics," *Annals of Internal Medicine* 134, no. 1 (2001): 84.

99. Charon, "Narrative Medicine: Form, Function, and Ethics," 9.

100. Thompson, "The Applicability of Narrative Ethics," 192.

101. Howard Spiro, "Empathy: An Introduction," in *Empathy and the Practice of Medicine,* ed. Howard Spiro, Mary Curnen, Enid Peschel, and Deborah St. James (New Haven, CT: Yale University Press, 1993).

102. Cassell, *The Nature of Suffering: And the Goals of Medicine,* 232

103. Charon, *Narrative Medicine: Honoring the Stories of Illness,* 190.

104. Ronald Andiman, "A Physician's Response to the Midrashic Invitation." William Cutter, *Midrash & Medicine: Healing Body and Soul in the Jewish Interpretive Tradition* (Woodstock, VT: Jewish Lights Pub., 2011), 97–104.

105. N. Guéguen, S. Meineri, and V. Charles-Sire, "Improving Medication Adherence by Using Practitioner Nonverbal Techniques: A Field Experiment on the Effect of Touch," *Journal of Behavioral Medicine* 33, no. 6 (2010): 466.

106. Michael White and David Epston, *Narrative Means to Therapeutic Ends* (New York: Norton, 1990), 3.

107. Ricoeur, *Time and Narrative,* vol. 3.

108. Arthur W. Frank, *The Wounded Storyteller: Body, Illness, and Ethics* (Chicago: University of Chicago Press, 1995).

109. Ibid., 7. Frank builds on social theory and post-structural philosophy to make claims about the narrative self.
110. Kathlyn Conway, *Beyond Words: Illness and the Limits of Expression* (Albuquerque: University of New Mexico Press, 2013a).
111. Conway, *Beyond Words*, 1.
112. Frank, *The Wounded Storyteller: Body, Illness, and Ethics*, 5.

Chapter 2

Narrative Identity and Practice in the Hospice Model of Care

Ricoeur's work on selfhood has specific applications for end-of-life care, and particularly for clinicians working with patients using methods in narrative medicine. In *Oneself as Another*, based on the Gifford Lectures he gave at the University of Edinburgh in 1986, Ricoeur examines the relationship between identity and selfhood and revisits the concept of narrative identity that he had previously addressed in his *Time and Narrative* series. In *Oneself as Another*, Ricoeur offers a counterpoint to the Cartesian cogito (I think; therefore, I am) as constitutive of identity based on the singular and first-person, "I." He situates himself between a positive conception of identity (the cogito) and a negative conception of identity (the empty, shattered, no-self). Instead of maintaining an exclusive focus on cognitive selfhood, Ricoeur maintains that selfhood has individual components—where a person attests to a narrative of selfhood, as well as social components—where others experience a person, and thereby create their own narrative of another based on this experience. As he notes in *Oneself as Another*, "Whole sections of my life are part of the history of others—of my parents, my friends, my companions in work and leisure."[1] Our lives are social and interconstitutive. For Ricoeur, we are both agents, who deliberate, act, and take responsibility for our actions, and we are acted upon by outside forces beyond the purview of our agency. Individuals are perceived and experienced by others and this interaction does not carry with it the certainty of identity the Cartesian cogito assumes. Nevertheless, selfhood can be understood, in part, by sameness over time.

For Ricoeur, identity and selfhood exist in a dialectical relationship with each other. A person changes over time, but there is also continuity in selfhood. He uses the terms idem and ipse to describe this dialectic between sameness over time (idem) and change over time (ipse/ipseity). The experience of aging reflects this dialectic. One experiences sameness over time—being the same physical, numerical self, while concurrently having awareness of how one's selfhood has changed over time, an experience of variability within continuity. For clinicians working with family members of patients with dementia, Ricoeur's dialectic of sameness-variability speaks about the grief and confusion experienced by family members who perceive the same person in front of them, who looks the same as they did before their cognitive decline, but the person in front of them has no memory of the family members or has a confused understanding of their relationship. This experience of the family member of a person with dementia reflects the dynamic between sameness over time and variations in selfhood. The strong Cartesian cogito offers the comfort of certainty, but what patients and family members actually experience calls this certainty into question. Ricoeur offers an understanding of selfhood that includes continuity as well as change over time, a model that is closer to the experience of health care patients and their family members.

Ricoeur's work on identity serves as a resource for understanding these existential crises. Who am I if I, the caregiver of the family, become dependent and have to be cared for? Who am I if I lose my ability to speak, reason, or remember? Who am I as I change over time? Questions of identity are connected with questions of social value and individual self-worth. Ricoeur recognized that there are elements of human existence that are consciously willed and those that we have limited control over. We act as agents in our lives, but we are also at the mercy of much that is out of our control. For instance, we do not choose where we are born, the families we are born into, our genetic makeup, or the traumatic events that occur in our lives. Additionally, there are elements to our narrative identity that blur with fiction; we are not necessarily reliable narrators of our own lived experience. His view on narrative identify diverges from Alasdair MacIntyre's approach—the "narrative unity of a life"—in that Ricoeur wants to emphasize the features of narrative selfhood that are constructed rather than directly recounted. He writes, "As for the notional of the narrative unity of a life, it must be seen as an unstable mixture of fabulation and actual experience."[2] Ricoeur gives the example of the beginning of life and the end of life as episodes that cannot be fully known or objectively narrated.[3]

In Ricoeur's view, humans have agency and freedom, but also experience conditions of existence that are out of their control; in *Oneself as Another*, he uses the language of passivity to describe this dimension of human experience. He identifies three interrelated categories of passivity: the physical, relational, and the individual. Physically, bodies are vulnerable to time, to illness, and death. Relationally, we cannot control or fully access how we are perceived by others or how they relate to us. On the individual level, there are aspects of our selves that are hidden and undetermined. Through aging, through the loss of physical and mental function, through loss and grief, one can experience one's existence as beholden to that which is outside of our control or understanding. One's self is then experienced as impossible to know fully and with certainty, and is instead experienced as distinct from one's known self, the way one would encounter another. Ricoeur writes in the tenth study of *Oneself as Another*, in "What Ontology in View?" that "otherness [is] at the heart of selfhood."[4]

The social nature of human identity and experience is central to Ricoeur's understanding of personhood and is the linchpin of his ethics. In the seventh study in *Oneself as Another*, "The Self and the Ethical Aim" Ricoeur builds on Aristotle's definition of ethics, as an aim for the "good life," grounded in praxis, to a more social view, defining what he calls the "ethical intention" as "aiming for the good life, with and for others, in just institutions."[5] Ricoeur offers a mediation between Aristotle's normative claims about what constitutes ethical relationships with others, examining Aristotle's example of friendship and reciprocity, and the views of Levinas, in which ethical demands are wholly initiated by others. He maintains that there is a giving-receiving dialectic at play in relationships, even in relationships of caregiving.[6]

Ricoeur's perspective on identity reflects the view of patient identity underlying the hospice model of care. For Ricoeur, identity is incarnational, social, narratival, and existential.[7] Similarly, in the hospice model of care, a patient is understood to be embodied, living in a relational context, with an individual story to tell and a spiritual or religious mode of being. What Ricoeur adds to the concept of patient identity for end-of-life patients is the view of the changing self that nevertheless remains constant over time. He also offers a reflection on death and how to be present with those facing the end of life in his collection of works, *Living Up to Death*, published posthumously in 2005, that I examine in the concluding chapter of this text. In the current chapter, I describe the patient identity assumed in the hospice model of care and I detail two narrative practices common in end-of-life care, life review, and spiritual assessments.

PATIENT IDENTITY IN THE HOSPICE MODEL OF CARE

In 1967, Cicely Saunders formally established the hospice model of care for terminal patients with the opening of St. Christopher's Hospice in London.[8] Previously, she worked with the Irish Sisters of Charity caring for terminal patients and spending time listening to their experiences and learning what care meant for them. Saunders observed that for many patients at the end of life, there was a deep need for companionship and personal attention beyond the medical. She recognized that care for terminal patients is multi-dimensional and includes attending to the patient's personal, social, and spiritual concerns, in addition to their medical needs. With this insight, she developed St. Christopher's Hospice as an intentionally religious space, designing the hospice with the chapel at the center of the building. Florence Wald, nurse and Dean of the Yale School of Nursing, after hearing Saunders speak and working with her in London, established the Connecticut Hospice in 1974, the first of its kind in the United States.[9] Hospice in the United States is a model of end-of-life care, often residence-based, for patients with a prognosis of six months or less to live. The goals of care address physical, spiritual, and psychosocial dimensions of patient identity. Pain management is a central feature of the hospice approach to care, and Saunders's definition of pain expands to include experiences of pain that are more than just physiological, observing that the end of life can be an experience of great pain for individuals and family members on a personal, social, and existential level. Her claims about the many dimensions of pain led to the Medicare requirement for hospices to include psychosocial support, volunteer presence, and spiritual and religious professionals to meet with patients and family members as part of the standard plan of care.

Hospice is a patient-centered model of care offering tailored treatment for an individual patient. Though patient-centered, the model of care is not individualistic, but is by nature relational, relying on those in some relationship to the patient to provide ongoing care including physical care such as feeding and bathing the patient, as well as nonclinical medical care such as providing medication when ordered by the medical directory or needed by the patient. In fact, one cannot enroll in hospice as an individual. Because hospice provides only episodic rather than continuous care, to be accepted as a hospice patient in the United States, one has to have full-time caregivers, either paid caregivers or unpaid caregivers in some form of relationship to the patient. While this model can be seen as limited considering that for many patients having caregivers is a luxury, there is nevertheless a relational component to this model of care that stands in contrast to the individualistic model of care provided by the biomedical model as it exists today. Hospice recognizes that total self-sufficiency may be an ideal for some, but the majority of individuals who are ill cannot care for themselves and the effects of the patient's illness affect the entire family rather than just the patient alone.

Underlying the hospice framework of care for terminal patients is an understanding of patient identity that expands beyond biological reductionism, often connected with the biomedical model of care, in which the patient's physical body is the focus of clinical attention.[10] In hospice, the patient is assumed to have medical, psychosocial, and spiritual needs. Though autonomy remains key to patient rights in hospice, the patient is viewed as interdependent and as having social needs which, if left unattended to, can be a source of unmanaged pain.[11] As pain management is central to the hospice philosophy of care, techniques used to address all forms of pain, including but expanding beyond its physical manifestations, are employed in the interest of total patient care.

CICELY SAUNDERS AND THE CONCEPT OF TOTAL PAIN

Cicely Saunders established the hospice model of care in response to three deficiencies she observed in the medical model of care for dying patients. The first concerns comprehensive pain management. Attending closely to patients and drawing on their first-person reports in her research, she identified a pattern of inadequate pain control for the dying. Saunders recognized that pain is not merely an event or a series of events, but for many terminal patients, pain is experienced as a state of being in which they are "held captive."[12] In her text *Living with Dying: The Management of Terminal Disease*, she noted that patients voiced their symptoms to clinicians but nevertheless continued to receive partial treatment.[13]

The legacy of her critique of pain control for the dying can be seen today in the attention given to comprehensive pain management, particularly by pharmacists and clinicians working in hospice and palliative care. Hospice physician Dr. Ira Byock maintains that all physical pain can be successfully treated medically.[14] This is not to say that pain is fully treated—Byock will be the first to say it is not—only to say that it can be if clinicians make this their goal.[15] The work of Saunders combined with the confidence of physicians and pharmacists that pain can be fully treated can assure patients (or the general population) that they will not have to die in pain. Dying in pain remains one of the top fears of individuals when they consider their deaths.

Saunders's second concern also relates to pain management for terminal patients. Saunders recognized that not all pain manifests physically—pain can have an inward dimension and be oriented to emotional, social, and spiritual matters. She coined the term "total pain" to describe how pain is experienced three-dimensionally, in body, mind, and spirit.[16] The different manifestations of pain call for a wide net of identification and treatment measures, transcending a pain management approach devoted entirely to the physical body. Yet, pain management for nonphysical pain such as spiritual or emotional distress does not necessarily call for palliation; in many such cases, direct inquiry into the sources of a person's psychosocial or spiritual distress provides relief and a sense of recognition. Allowing the patient to examine his or her suffering, rather than attempting to assuage this pain, can offer succor to a patient whose pain may be avoided by others because the intractability of the person's pain discomfits them. Mere recognition that a person is in emotional pain can provide relief for those in distress. Also, physical, spiritual, social, and emotional experiences of pain interconnect and impact each other; Saunders observed that after receiving spiritual and psychosocial attention to their concerns patients reported less pain.

Largely due to the research and advocacy of Cicely Saunders, medical treatment no longer relies solely on pharmacological treatment or the physician's independent judgment of the patient's experience of pain. Numerical pain scales (giving a number for the level of one's pain), face scales (choosing a face on the scale whose expression matches one's experience), and other forms of naming the subjective experience of pain are now used by clinicians and caregivers.[17] Supplemental therapies are also increasingly used to mitigate pain for patients—massage, music therapy, and pet therapy, while still considered alternative modes of pain control, exist in the array of pain management possibilities available today. Saunders work on total pain accelerated medical interest in pain management and turned needed attention to extrapharmacological forms of pain control for patients. Medical and nonmedical forms of symptom management are not in conflict in her comprehensive view of patient care; her primary motive is to attend to what works to mitigate pain and suffering for patients, regardless of the source.

Finally, Saunders emphasized recognition of the dignity of terminal patients, recognizing that the treatment of patients calls for compassion and respect. She maintained that research on end-of-life care was a crucial part of demonstrating respect for the dying.[18] Accordingly, she called for new attention to pharmacological treatments for pain and prioritized patient comfort over a clinician's fear of opiate addition.[19] Saunders emphasized a shift in medical epistemology, envisioning a model of care devoted to the treatment of pain in all of its manifestations. Her normative vision for medical care for end-of-life patients led to increased attention given to pain management for dying patients receiving clinical care and encouraged a renewed focus on the spiritual and psychosocial aspects of end-of-life care.

PAIN AND PATIENT IDENTITY

The hospice philosophy offers an alternative approach to patient identity that expands beyond the biological reductionism found in medical models, particularly models in which clinicians focus their care exclusively on the body. In contrast, the hospice model as designed by Saunders conceives of patient identity in three parts, including an inward, personal dimension, a social identity formed by multiple strands of relationality, and, for many, a sense of identity that includes a sense of the spiritual and a connection to organized religion, be this active engagement or estrangement. Paralleling this view of identity, the concept of pain in hospice includes recognition of personal suffering, relational tension, and spiritual or existential distress. The hospice team is structured so that team members coordinate individual care for patients by creating a tailored plan of care that addresses medical, personal, social, and spiritual needs, with specific attention given to the sources of a patient's pain. Whereas the clinical goal in hospice is to manage physical pain so that the patient is comfortable, comfort is not necessarily a goal for the personal, social, and spiritual experiences of pain. Narrative practices such as life review can move a patient to consider ways in which they fell short of their hopes and expectations for themselves and thus be a contributing factor for an increase in emotional pain. The process can disinter painful memories for patients or can bring into sharp relief the dysfunction that exists within families. Overall, the goals of pain management within hospice differ depending on type of pain a patient experiences: for physical pain the goal is comfort, but for the nonphysical dimensions of pain, the goal may be to allow the pain to be identified, named, and examined without an expectation of therapeutic outcomes.

There are various sources of emotional, social, and spiritual pain for those facing the end of life. In addition to the emotional impact of receiving a terminal diagnosis, a person can be grieving an accumulation of losses: loss of health, abilities, and independence, future possibilities, relationships, loss of a job or the ability to engage in personal hobbies, and the losses of valued markers of identity or experience. There may be the radical fear that one has passed on an inheritable terminal illness to one's children. Self-blame and condemnation can create anguish for patients who believe they brought their illness on themselves due to behaviors or lack of faith. One of the key differences between the pain of despair and physical manifestations of pain is that the former cannot be easily assessed and efficiently treated. Physical pain can be reported by the patient, but can also be observed by others in the form of clenched hands, a furrowed brow, sounds of discomfort, wincing, and agitation. Inward pain, though it also has physical manifestations through observable bodily tension, is primarily communicated through language. Meeting with a chaplain can prompt conversations about personal distress that may not occur with medical caregivers. However, it is imperative that clinicians learn when to make appropriate referrals for patients in despair. Failure to diagnose and make proper referrals for patients in emotional or spiritual pain signals an ethically problematic neglect of their comprehensive well-being because it does not attend to their total pain.

Patients in emotional or spiritual distress can trigger a sense of impotence for clinicians. Trained to be diagnosticians and healers, the professional abilities of medial clinicians reach a limit-point for patients in despair because as there is no standardized treatment plan for a patient's personal anguish. Also, when patients are angry about their health predicaments or medical issues, they may lash out at caregivers and clinicians which can lead others to avoid them or spend as little time as possible facing their distress. Nevertheless, difficult patients deserve comprehensive care and sufficient attention despite their presentation, particularly as their exacting state of being may be a symptom of unrecognized emotional pain or physical pain. When a patient is experiencing emotional or existential distress, having a conversation about their concerns can provide comfort and relief. Clinicians trained in methods in narrative medicine are able to listen to patients as they process their fears and personal concerns.

LONELINESS AS A MANIFESTATION OF PAIN

One of the elements of total pain identified by Saunders is the pain that comes from isolation for end-of-life patients. Because of the taboo against death and dying in the United States, and even the sense that death and misfortune can be contagious, terminal patients often go unvisited by friends and family members. Though many patients receive physical caregiving, they may receive little social stimulation via conversation or other forms of engaged activities. Mobility can be limited for terminal patients, restricting them to their place of residence. Some patients are bedbound and placed in rooms in low traffic parts of homes or hospital wings, receiving little human interaction. Though she did not use the language of "quality of life" common today, a term that can include social dimensions of patient experience, Saunders recognized the distress that comes from limited relationality and considered it worthy of attention in a patient's plan of care.

The attenuation of relationships for patients at the end of life can result in a near-solitary existence; even if patients reside in assisted living facilities they may experience isolation among others. Hospice addresses this form of social pain by offering volunteer companionship to patients, a visitor that comes in a nonprofessional role without even a plan of care. Though there is no set plan of care, a volunteer may engage a patient in a dialogical process of retrospection called "life review." Due to its social quality, the process can assuage the pain that comes from isolation and loneliness for patients at the end of life. Life review represents a narrative-based practice that clinicians can use with patients, one that reflects the Ricoeurian view of selfhood as narratival and social.

LIFE REVIEW AND NARRATIVE PRACTICES IN THE HOSPICE MODEL OF CARE

"Life review" is the term for a narrative process of reminiscence for hospice patients, often facilitated by a volunteer companion. Volunteers are a required part of the care team in the hospice model of care. In addition to skilled nursing care, Medicare requires that 5 percent of patient hours be provided by volunteers.[20] If a patient or a patient's caregivers accept volunteer support, volunteer time is then ordered by the medical director on the patient's official plan of care. When volunteers visit patients, their primary goal is to provide social support for patients or respite for caregivers. Because they accompany patients in a nonclinical role, a patient may feel free to speak with more openness than if a professional caregiver were there, working with the patient toward a specific goal of care. When a patient accepts a volunteer for social support, engaging in life review is one of the activities that can be available for them. Life review reflects the dialogical nature of the clinical encounter with hospice patients and their caregivers. The process of life review includes self-reflection based on a retrospective view of one's life. The process of life review can have either a positive or a negative valence depending on the patient's perspective.

How Chaplains and Spiritual Counselors Utilize Life Review

When a patient is admitted to hospice, Medicare guidelines require a comprehensive care plan to be established within the first five days of admission.[21] The role of the hospice chaplain can be conceptualized as a spiritual or religious counselor available for the patient and those close to the patient to discuss their beliefs or values; an assessment of the patient's preferences to discuss their concerns with a spiritual counselor is one of the required measures for assessment along with an assessment of pain, dyspnea, and bowel responses to medication.[22] The inclusion of a spiritual assessment early in the patient's admission, if the patient chooses one, supports Cicely Saunders's claim that spiritual pain is a dimension of total pain. If the goal of hospice is comfort and the management of total pain for patients, this then would require professional attention given to emotional, social, and spiritual pain, alongside the attention given to physical pain. Physical pain includes nausea and agitation and other forms of physical discomfort. Regarding clinical goals of care, the major distinction between the approach to physical pain as distinct from spiritual pain is that physical pain is meant to be fully treated, if possible and if preferred by the patient. Some patients prefer not to experience the sedating effects of opioid medication, choosing the benefit of clarity over the experience of pain. However, the goals of care for spiritual counselors are not necessarily focused on the elimination of pain. Rather, when physical pain is sufficiently managed, the patient then has the capability to examine one's life, via processes like life review or dignity therapy, common interventions for chaplains.[23] Such reflections may actually be a source of emotional, social, or spiritual pain for the patient, but the chaplain's role is to work with the patient as the patient examines these concerns, rather than attempting to end or solve this pain.

For Cicely Saunders, physical pain must be managed so that other forms of pain can be attended to. The goal is not to eliminate suffering in its entirety. The goal is to eliminate physical pain so that a patient can encounter their suffering (their emotional, social, religious, and existential suffering) and deal with it on their terms. A sense of peace and contentment can occur, but it is not the primary goal of care. This is particularly the case for spiritual counselors as compared to social workers because concerns regarding guilt, judgment, and confession often have religious tinges. Engaging in life review with a spiritual or religious counselor will thus unearth concerns with God's judgment, punishment in the afterlife, guilt, penance, and lament; language that is less likely to be used with a secular counselor. By acknowledging these areas of pain and suffering with a chaplain or spiritual counselor, the patient may experience relief or resolution of their spiritual and existential distress, but this is not a certain outcome. A study on the nature of spiritual pain experienced by palliative patients found that patients wanted a chaplain to listen, provide a sense of presence for them, and accompany them as they navigate their concerns.[24] Life review with chaplains can be initiated formally or occur spontaneously as a patient reflects on their sources of comfort and pain.

For some patients, the dialogical process of life review can lead to emotional distress, a dimension of psychosocial spiritual pain, or what Saunders calls "total pain." Chaplains can provide therapeutic presence for patients in their distress as they talk through regrets, disappointments, fears, hopelessness, and other forms of emotional and existential concern. Because the interaction between chaplain and patient is fundamentally conversational in nature, methods in narrative medicine can be utilized to deepen the clinical, pastoral encounter. Learning to be a close reader of text, to be attuned to nuance and detail, to be aware of the inner existence of another person, these are all skills developed through methods in narrative medicine, and they are skills that have a one-to-one parallel to the chaplain-patient encounter. Through narrative methods that teach attention to detail, a chaplain in a hospital setting can learn to enter a room alert to signifiers of religiosity on the part of the patient. Do they have a copy of the Torah, prayer beads, statues or religiously themed greeting cards displayed? Such items can be invitations to learn more about a patient's religious identity. Narrative methods that teach a clinician how to be aware of a person's interior life are also valuable for chaplains. Learning to be a close reader of texts involves an awareness of the interiority of another person, through the form of a character, and a chaplain can draw on narrative methods to practice increasing his or her awareness of the inner life of a patient.

With hospice patients in particular, many concerns of the patient are non-medical in nature. A patient may be concerned with how his or her children will cope with the loss of a parent and worry about how they will do on their own without parental guidance. A patient may fear being institutionalized at a nursing facility or dying in the hospital. Many patients fear dying in pain. The anxiety that comes with shortness of breath is one that can be treated medically, through the use of medications that calm the breathing reflex, but it is also an experience that can be addressed through nonpharmacological means, such as through deep breathing exercises that can be done with a chaplain. The experience of prayer can have a calming influence on patients. Prayer is an act in which a chaplain engages in an interpretive, narrative act. The chaplain takes into account the scene in which the patient is found and names the exterior and interior dimensions of this experience, calling on God, however understood by the patient, to be present with the patient.

Narrative Medicine and the Role of the Chaplain

Because patients can experience emotional and existential distress when facing a health crisis or life events like birth or death, having a person there to sit beside them and listen as they process the contours of their new world can be instrumental in the therapeutic process. Hospices in the United States are required by Medicare to have chaplains or spiritual counselors on their care teams, available to patients and family members for spiritual support and bereavement care. Hospitals similarly are mandated to offer support for the spiritual care needs of patients and families, though hospitals do not necessarily have the collaborative approach to care modeled by hospices in which chaplains sit alongside nurses, physicians, and social workers in weekly interdisciplinary team meetings to discuss a patient's plan of care. In these meetings, clinicians discuss a patient's pain, anxiety, and emotional or spiritual distress and work jointly to determine the appropriate plan of care for the patient. When hospital clinicians are attuned to the extra-medical needs of patients, such as the experience of spiritual or existential distress, they can then make referrals within the hospital system for chaplains to attend to the patient's concerns.

Chaplains working in a health care context often describe their role as that of a listening presence for patients and family members as they navigate the complex terrain of medical treatment and the fear and uncertainty provoked by a health care crisis. From the shock of an unexpected diagnosis that interrupts a person's life plan to the swallowing experience of grief when facing the death of a loved one, a person's experience in the hospital cannot be limited or reduced the merely medical. Evidence-based medicine seeks to generalize human experience, and this model works well in a diagnostic model of care, but a person experiences the fallout of a medical crisis in ways that vary and that require time, trust, and relationality to share. A physician is there to make a medical judgment based on the patient's needs; a chaplain, in contrast, is there as a nonjudgmental listening presence, there to receive the patient's own interpretation of his or her experience. Chaplains also serve as liaison between the medical clinicians and the patient's family members, particularly in trauma situations. Also chaplains can link a patient to a patient's religious community, thereby increasing social support and affirming Ricoeur's view of the social dimensions of human nature.

The work chaplains engage in is fundamentally dialogical and interpretive. In *Lost in Translation: The Chaplain's Role in Health Care*, the authors describe chaplains as "translators," able to assist health care providers in caring for the patient in a personalized way.[25] They note, "While medical professionals focus on patients' medical conditions, chaplains seek to read the whole person, asking questions about what people's lives are like outside of the hospital, what they care about most, and where they find joy and support in the world. Chaplains offer a supportive presence that serves to remind patients and caregivers that people are more than just their medical conditions or their current collection of concerns." The role of chaplains includes, but is not limited to, spiritual and religious care for a patient. In many cases, patients are working with questions of identity or existential distress, subjects that fall outside neat categories of spiritual or religious care, but nevertheless call for therapeutic attention in a health care context. Undoubtedly, many physicians have the clinical communication skills necessary to work with patients in emotional or existential distress, but in a health care context, chaplains are the ones who have the time to meet with patients as they address their concerns, a process in which the clinical goals of efficiency and precision do not necessarily apply.

In hospice, chaplains and clinical caregivers work together on a health care team. Clinical caregivers identify and strive to treat physical manifestations of pain and discomfort. As a support service complementing medical care, chaplaincy involves accompanying patients as they experience spiritual, social, and existential pain. Fear, regret, and loneliness cannot be treated medically; they must be addressed on a personal level. The dimensions of passivity that Ricoeur describes emerge in the clinical encounter between chaplains, patients, and patients' family members. Patients describe the ways in which their bodies have changed over time, how their relationships have strengthened or attenuated, and how they feel frustrated when recognizing the limits of their ability to remember who they were or where they are. Patients experiencing cognitive decline nevertheless have moments of lucidity when they recognize that they cannot remember details of their lives.

Chaplains working in a health care context face challenges that can be addressed through narrative methods in their clinical education. Interactions between chaplains and patients are often dialogical in nature due to the conversational nature of spiritual assessments.

From the Joint Commission, formerly the Joint Commission on Accreditation of Healthcare Organizations (JCAHO), the following are examples of questions that can be asked to make spiritual assessments:

- Who or what provides the patient with strength and hope?
- Does the patient use prayer in their life?
- How does the patient express their spirituality?
- How would the patient describe their philosophy of life?
- What type of spiritual/religious support does the patient desire?
- What is the name of the patient's clergy, ministers, chaplains, pastor, rabbi?
- What does suffering mean to the patient?
- What does dying mean to the patient?
- What are the patient's spiritual goals?
- Is there a role of church/synagogue in the patient's life?
- How does your faith help the patient cope with illness?
- How does the patient keep going day after day?
- What helps the patient get through this health care experience?
- How has illness affected the patient and his/her family?[26]

Such questions are likely to prompt a longer conversation with patients and having clinicians, including health care chaplains, available, who are trained in methods in narrative medicine create the space for attentive dialogue with patients, giving them sufficient time to reflect on and discuss their pain in its different manifestations, physical, psychological, social, and spiritual.

Bringing Methods in Narrative Medicine to Clinical Pastoral Education

Methods in narrative medicine provide an avenue for practicing close listening skills for chaplains. The central premise in narrative medicine is that learning to be a close reader of texts can teach a clinician how to be attentive to patients in the clinical encounter. Because clinical pastoral education (CPE) involves group debriefing sessions, these sessions can be used to discuss and analyze a shared text such as a short story. Engaging in this exercise will encourage students to be aware of the experience of others, through encounters with fictional characters, and group discussions will reveal the multiplicity of interpretations that can emerge from the reading of a shared text. In addition to developing listening skills, the variety of interpretations chaplain residents will encounter can be a segue to teaching about family systems in a health care context. Too often, education in health care is oriented toward care for an individual patient, when the practice of health care involves attending to the social context of the patient—the patient's family and religious community, for example.

To become board certified in chaplaincy in the United States, a student must participate in an educational program called clinical pastoral education, an immersive model of education often based in acute-care hospital settings. Clinical pastoral education has no standard curriculum and assumes the experience of working as a chaplain under supervision provides sufficient education for professional chaplains. Some programs offer educational sessions called "didactics," but there is no core-curriculum in CPE consistent among programs. Scholars such as Alexander Tartaglia see this model as limited and have called for a more standardized model of education to ensure that chaplains complete a residency program that addresses the competencies required for board certification.[27]

Listening is a common intervention and, though many aspiring chaplains already demonstrate strong listening skills, there is nevertheless reason to intentionally train chaplains in communication skills and active listening as this form of engagement is the linchpin of clinical pastoral care. Patients in acute-care settings can be in critical emotional and existential distress and they deserve be cared for by individuals trained in therapeutic practices. Chaplains can also benefit from training in how to respond to patients in trauma, as many chaplains are on call in emergency departments. Another component of listening skills applies to providing emotional and spiritual care to the hospital staff who may be suffering from multiple losses and workplace stress. The immersive educational model of CPE as it exists today can be supplemented by a skills-based educational model for chaplain residents.

Bereavement Care and Social Selfhood

In addition to the medical, psychosocial, and spiritual care provided to patients enrolled in hospice, the Medicare guidelines require that family members and friends have the option of receiving bereavement counseling services prior to the patient's death and following the death for a minimum of one year.[28] Bereavement care for family and friends begins before the patient's death to ensure that the counseling services provided are tailored to the individual person, rather than being a carte blanche kind of therapy.[29]

Typically, bereavement needs of those close to the terminal patient are assessed by the social worker or chaplain on the interdisciplinary team who then communicate their clinical opinion to the bereavement counselor during the weekly team meetings.[30] Such an inclusive model of clinical care recognizes that a patient does not exist as an isolated, self-sufficient, self-defined entity, but that the majority of individuals exist in a matrix of relationships, positive and negative. The self in hospice is perceived fundamentally as a social self, aligning with Ricoeur's view of selfhood.

A concept of the social self proves important in those cases in which the patient is referred to hospice late in their disease progression. In situations of late referrals (understood here to mean referrals that occur seven days or less before death occurs), which according to the 2016 Medicare guidelines were over 35 percent of patients receiving hospice care, attention shifts to prioritizing medical care for the patient with specific focus on pain management and arranging details regarding the context of care.[31] As a patient transitions, there can be less interest in the outside world and less energy to engage in the give and take of conversation and social interaction. The patient turns inward and may not speak or show signs of external awareness of others in the last days of life. In the context of a late referral where the patient is close to transitioning, the focus for the care team is less on the psychosocial or spiritual needs of the patient and more on ensuring that the patient's physical pain is appropriately managed and that they are comfortable.

In the event of a late referral to hospice, there may not be time for the chaplain, volunteer, or counselor to engage in a deliberate form of life review with patients. However, this does not mean that life review did not occur. In cases in which a terminal diagnosis is known by the patient, perhaps intuitively, they can begin to process their life and reflect on their choices, opportunities taken or missed, and relationships with their family and friends. The hospice team may not hear these accounts, but the person's companions often do in the period preceding hospice enrollment. Through bereavement counseling provided by hospice, the bereaved have an opportunity to communicate the individual's life review narrative in remembrance of the person, demonstrating the social dimensions of narrative selfhood. Social or secondary life review accounts reflect the variety of emotional responses that occur in relationships, not just positive reminiscences. According to Hooyman and Kramer, "An active confrontation with the loss—through rage, anger, and the honest expression of sorrow—is widely assumed to be necessary for deliverance from the past, as it requires recognizing all facets of the loss."[32] There can be awareness on the part of the bereaved of the hopes or goals of the patient that were not realized because of their diagnosis. For parents experiencing the death of child, there is reflection on the life that might have been.[33] The proximity to the truth, or sense of self perceived by the patient as distinct from how it is perceived and described by the bereaved, matters less than the therapeutic value of the process.

ATTENDING TO THE RELIGIOUS DIMENSION OF HUMAN EXPERIENCE

In addition to viewing patient identity as narratival and social, hospice recognizes the religious dimension of human experience as existential and spiritual. Though hospices today are unlikely to have an overtly religious mission or vision statement like St. Christopher's, there continues to be recognition of the role religion and spirituality have in the provision of care.[34] The Joint Commission requires that hospitals attend to the spiritual and religious needs of patients. The Joint Commission does not specify or mandate how this attention should manifest, but nevertheless there is institutional recognition of the place of religion in a medical context.[35] Abiding by a patient-centered mission involves approaching patient care as a multi-dimensional task, rather than limiting patient care to the biological. Recognition of the role of religion and spirituality in medical care continues to grow, due in large part to the advocacy and scholarship of physicians interested in the subject, particularly Christina Puchalski and Daniel Sulmasy. Codeveloper of FICA, a commonly used spiritual assessment tool, Puchalski advocates for routine spiritual assessments when physicians take patient histories; she strives to normalize conversations that take into account the religious and spiritual dimensions of patients. Though JCAHO maintains in their diversity statement that physicians have an obligation to respect a patient's religion, Puchalski takes this obligation further to include the recognition and assessment of a patient's individual needs as an aspect of clinical care.[36]

In addition to expanding the scope of what should be included in the clinical encounter, Puchalski's vision has a pedagogical focus. She maintains that all medical students should have education available that addresses the religious and spiritual component of patient care, and that comprehensive, patient-centered care for all patients includes recognition of the patient's world of meaning; as it is now, palliative care is the only domain of medicine that specifically includes attention to religion and spirituality in the goals of care.[37] Her advocacy has been instrumental in the expansion of medical school curricula that includes religion and spirituality, not merely as a domain of the medical humanities, but as central to clinical care for patients.[38] Her concept of health extends beyond physical wellness, instead cohering with the World Health Organization's definition of health as the "dynamic state of complete physical, mental, spiritual, and social well-being and not just the absence of disease or infirmity."[39] She maintains that comprehensive care for patients includes recognition of the spiritual and religious dimensions of their lives. Physicians often hesitate to inquire about a patient's religiosity because they do not feel adequately trained in the study of religion, hence her promotion of curricula on religion in clinical training.

Scholarship by Daniel Sulmasy similarly addresses the need to attend to a patient's spiritual and religious identity, particularly for patients at the end of life. Sulmasy, a physician and former Franciscan friar, notes that patients prefer that their physicians inquire about the subject in the clinical encounter, regardless of the physician's identification as religious.[40] There is no need to abide by a strict secularism in the medical context, as "the artificial neutrality of enforced secularism inevitably leads to a discussion that is conceptually impoverished, lacking the language to address the existential questions of suffering in ways that are meaningful to the patient."[41] In fact, Sulmasy maintains that physicians have a moral obligation to actively inquire about a patient's spiritual and religious identity, both because potential sources of support and meaning can go untapped.[42] To the question of whether or not it is the role of the clinician to inquire about a patient's spiritual concerns, he responds, "[I]f physicians and other healthcare professionals have sworn to treat patients to the best of their ability and judgment, and the best care treats patients as whole persons, then to treat patients in a way that ignores the fundamental meaning that the patient sees in suffering, healing, life, and death is to treat patients superficially and to fall short of the best ability and judgment."[43] For Sulmasy, a clinical posture based on respect for patients as persons includes recognition of the spiritual and religious dimensions of their identity.

Sulmasy worries that a patient's spiritual distress may be neglected by physicians hesitant to engage in conversations about religion and spirituality in the clinical encounter. However, he recognizes that while religiosity can provide comfort for some patients, this does not hold true for all.[44] Manifestations of religious coping in response to illness can be both negative and positive, making the need for clinical assessment of how the patient understands the function of religion and spirituality in his or her life all the more crucial. On the negative side, patients may feel guilt, anxiety, fear, and denial as a result of their religious or theological framework.[45] Positively, religious coping can provide a sense of meaning, value, and connection for patients, in addition to linking a patient to a supportive community.[46] Though Sulmasy does note the medical benefits of belief and a sense of the transcendent, his reason for promoting conversations about spirituality and religion in the clinical encounter does not spring from an interest in medical efficacy. He does not believe the sacred should, or can, be limited or instrumentalized to the medical benefits one may experience as a result of belief. Like Puchalski, Sulmasy does not believe a lack of religiosity of the part of the physician should preclude conversations about a patient's beliefs. Both Puchalski and

Sulmasy recognize that the professional capacity of physicians does not include pastoral care; consequently, they maintain that physicians make referrals to chaplains or the spiritual care department for specialized attention to religious and spiritual needs.[47]

RELIGION IN CLINICAL MEDICAL EDUCATION

Curricula designed to train clinicians in taking a spiritual history are becoming more common in medical education. In residency programs, clinicians may encounter more sustained exposure to spiritual care if there is an active spiritual care program in their internship environment. In addition to the patient-centered aspects of recognizing a patient's religious and spiritual identity, there is medical value in training a clinician to inquire about a patient's spiritual and religious history and identity. Patients often make medical decisions based on their religious framework, so the relationship between medicine and religion calls for clinical attention. Decisions regarding end-of-life care, resuscitation, reproductive decisions, autopsies, organ donation, pain management, and blood transfusions are just a few examples of when a patient's religious identity informs their decision-making. Patients may have some spiritual conflict that warrants further conversation about their spiritual well-being. Also, patients indicate that they want their clinicians to inquire about their spiritual or religious lives.[48] Cicely Saunders's recognition that the spiritual dimension of human identity relates to clinical care is not one that is limited to end-of-life care; however, the end of life is a unique time of religious reflection for many individuals and attention to this reflective activity is valuable in a medical context.

SPIRITUAL ASSESSMENTS AS AN EXAMPLE OF NARRATIVE PRACTICE

Because patients indicate that they would like their physicians to address their spiritual life, educational material regarding the subject is becoming more prominent in medical education. Christina Puchalski advocates for medical training that includes material on religion and spirituality, but mere exposure to models of spiritual care such as those taught in an introductory course does not ensure that a clinician has had adequate training in discerning when it is appropriate or inappropriate for the clinician to prompt a conversation about religion or make religious statements.[49] Various assessment tools exist that are designed to address a patient's spiritual and religious needs. Due to the open-ended and personal nature of the questions asked in spiritual assessment tools, these assessment tools are likely to lead to a clinical encounter structured on narrativity. The most commonly used assessment tools are FICA,[50] SPIRIT,[51] HOPE,[52] and the 7 × 7 model.[53] In general, the tools inquire about a patient's religious and spiritual identity, their connection to a religious social group, how their religion connects with how they understand why they are in the hospital, and how they would like their spiritual and religious needs to be addressed. The dialogical tools also assess whether or not religion is used as a positive or negative means of coping with illness and how they expect their religion to serve them in the future.

Gordon Allport, Harvard psychologist and, along with William James, one of the earliest social scientists to critically examine religiosity as a legitimate and nonpathological subject, offered a distinction with regard to approaches to religion that can be used to clarify how its role is understood in medicine. In his text, *The Individual and His Religion*, he distinguishes between intrinsic and extrinsic religiosity; intrinsic religiosity is how Allport describes religion as an end in and of itself in which a person internalizes religious values and extrinsic religiosity is more performative, a mode of religiosity that is used as a means to an end.[54] Allport in collaboration with Michael Ross developed one of the first assessments of religiosity, the Religious Orientation Scale, a precursor to the spiritual assessments that exist today.[55] The spiritual assessments used today specifically address the intrinsic and extrinsic religiosity of patients.[56] Additionally, much of the scholarship on religion and medicine concerns the religiosity of the patient, with some recognition of the ways attending to the religious and spiritual needs of patients can meet forms of extrinsic religiosity for clinicians (such as prayer in the clinical encounter). I submit that there is value in attending to the intrinsic religiosity of caregivers as well, a subject I address in the concluding section of this chapter.

There are two distinct benefits that result from addressing the religiosity of patients. First, a person can be reminded of how his or her religion understands human value. For instance, in the Christian tradition, a person's value does not come from extrinsic categories of worth (one's job, familial status, gender, social position, etc.). Rather, a person's value is fundamentally intrinsic, coming from being made in the image of God.[57] The second benefit concerns how life and death are framed. If the goal of life is not achievement or longevity but communion with God, the prospect of death can be less terrifying. Research shows that those who ascribe to religious belief are less likely to consider ending their lives prematurely through the means of physician-assisted suicide.[58] If death is considered to be a time of presence with the sacred, or a point on the journey toward presence with the sacred, a person may feel less alone and afraid to transition from life.

In addition to the theological support that can result from recognizing a patient's religiosity and prompting reminders of how the patient's religion understands human value and the event of death, there are medical reasons for inviting conversation about a patient's religiosity or spiritual identity. Patients can be connected with their communities of support and receive social stimulation through such religious networks; this is particularly valuable for patients who may not receive support from their families of origin. Additionally, there are religious and spiritual methods of pain management that can comfort patients when other means are insufficient. As religion focuses on healing rather than treatment or cure, religion can be especially valuable for those who are dying from a terminal disease where cure is not possible.

Critiques of Spiritual Assessments

Some scholars critique spiritual assessment tools for perpetuating a "checklist mentality" in care, one in which the patient is asked about their history in a cursory way just to meet the institution's assessment requirements. The underlying idea is that spiritual care is passively conforming to a medical model based on quantitative standards of care.[59] A similar critique is made of principlism in medical ethics, that the four principles of autonomy, beneficence, nonmaleficence, and justice become four categories that can be briefly considered, a cursory approach that can result in overlooking or ignoring other ethical issues that may arise in clinical care. As with principlism in medical ethics, spiritual assessments may appear to be simple heuristics used to document that a patient's concerns have been addressed; however, the communication tools often serve as prompts to deepen conversations about a patient's fears, concerns, or care preferences. Though in some cases they can be limited communication devices, based on the person using them or the context of their use, they are intended to be springboards to further dialogue or to serve as vehicles for making pastoral care referrals. The alternative to not using spiritual assessment tools, even when used in checklist fashion, is to risk neglecting a patient's spiritual and religious identity, one that often provides solace and social support during times of illness or medical need.

Those critical of spiritual assessment tools can overstate their case when they address their concerns exclusively to admission questionnaires or to quantitative standards. As described previously, not all tools are quantitative measures of spiritual needs; instead many of them are qualitative guides to open-ended discussion. It is worth noting, however, that the very questions asked in the standards do structure and in ways limit the conversation. When the conversation is primarily directed by the clinician based on set questions, the patient then becomes a passive recipient of attention rather than the agent in the conversation. The efficacy of the tool depends on the person inviting the conversation. When referrals to other spiritual caregivers are made, this allows greater opportunity for a patient to connect with someone he or she feels comfortable with. Ultimately, spiritual assessments are useful for identifying spiritual distress and the ways in which a patient's spiritual and religious identity can possibly shape their medical decisions. They also serve as methods of engaging in patient-centered care and provide an object of conversation for patients who may be radically socially isolated; this is especially true for those at the end of life. Critiques that the assessments are designed to quantify, control, or measure a patient's spiritual or religious identity fail to recognize that the value for the patient may differ from the institutional value of the assessments. Additionally, it is better for a patient's religious or spiritual identity to be recognized via a portable, generic tool such as one of the pneumonically named prompts, rather than the patient's religious and spiritual identity be neglected out of an overzealous fear of constricting the conversation. Furthermore, the religious and spiritual assessments are valuable in that they can keep the conversation focused on the patient's identity. The potential exists for a professional caregiver, especially for clinicians and chaplains in training, to speak about his or her own beliefs, thereby inappropriately controlling or influencing a patient due to the asymmetry of power involved in the relationship. Rather than being a flaw, the structured nature of established spiritual assessments such as HOPE, FICA, and SPIRIT then beneficially limits and directs the conversation to the patient's spiritual or religious identity.

DISTINCTION BETWEEN SPIRITUAL ASSESSMENTS AND LIFE REVIEW

Life review in hospice relates to spiritual assessments in the following ways. One, both are structured on a narrative presentation of the patient's experience that emerge in dialogical fashion. Additionally, both modalities of narration can elicit positive and negative responses in patients, reports of satisfaction and gratitude as well as reports of anger, sorrow, regret, and a sense of injustice. Both call on the patient to reflect on his or her individual life, taking into account the ways one has been formed by significant roles and relationships. In this sense, both models move beyond scientific medicine into the domain of humanistic care, highly oriented to the patient as person.

Spiritual assessments and life review are distinct in that spiritual assessments, though structured on open-ended questions, are goal-based and formalized though the use of specific questions, hence the frequent use of acronyms for spiritual assessments. The goal is to locate sources of spiritual and religious support for the patient and to identify any spiritual or religious distress the patient may have. Referrals to chaplains can then be made, and the chaplain can connect the patient with sources of support in the community or offer pastoral care and counseling for distress the patient or family may have. Whereas life review is supplemental to patient care, spiritual assessments are part of admission protocol in many hospitals, due to the Joint Commission's standards of spiritual assessment.

Questions of meaning, identity, and moral behavior can emerge in both forms of assessment. Even if the individual does not identify as religious, chances are high that religion shaped his or her formation, through schooling, political life, aesthetics, gender expectations, and so on. As Daniel Sulmasy notes, even those who are atheist or hostile to religion still demonstrate a relationship with religion and cannot claim that it plays no role in their lives. Comments related to forgiveness, regret, accomplishment, all can be interpreted from a religious framework. Additionally, a sense of fear that one did not live in a way that honored God is explicitly religious. Comments that concern being punished in death for what a person did or did not do in life are saturated in religiosity. In cases where individuals disclose their fear or terror being judged after they die, it is crucial to heed Margaret Mohrmann's admonition to be acutely aware of the impulse to try to "heal" or "fix" the person, to force a sense of closure on someone.[60] While a sense of peace and healing can occur, recognizing the source of this desire is necessary in the encounter with a dying patient. Is the patient the one interested in healing or is it the person facilitating dialogue? Mohrmann notes the danger of imposing one's own sense of justice or healing onto another person in an "imperialism of empathy."[61]

Life review has a retrospective focus more so than spiritual assessments, which are designed to identify immediate needs or resources of support. In life review, a patient considers the content of his or her life, turning toward how one lived rather than how one will live. In spiritual assessments, because they are done on patients who are not terminal, there can be more of a focus on the patient's present experience and on the patient's hopes for the future.

Both models allow a patient an opportunity to discuss types of pain that are nonmedical in nature. Elaine Scarry notes that pain limits communication and the understanding of others when it comes to another person's pain.[62] However, as Anne Jurecic suggests in *Illness as Narrative*, this radical inability to articulate one's pain can be overstated.[63] Jurecic maintains that there can be a shared experience of pain, and that the shared reality of pain can be experienced in vicarious ways, such as through literature and other modalities of narrative medicine. When a patient is allowed an opportunity to discuss pain with his or her caregiver, this allows for the possibility that the patient will be connected to resources that serve to address this pain, such as the possibility of a pastoral care referral.

The role of the patient's interlocutor provides another distinction between the two methods of discourse. Due largely to the advocacy of Christine

Puchalski, spiritual assessments are typically done by the physician as a feature of the patient's medical history. Research shows that patients would like their physicians to inquire about the religious and spiritual dimensions of their identities. Life review, on the other hand, is often engaged in with a volunteer companion or a family member, a dynamic less influenced by a hierarchical role structure. Clinicians may be constrained by organizational factors and have less time to listen patients reflect on concerns that are not immediately medical.

CONCLUSION

The hospice philosophy of patient care, as established by founder Cicely Saunders, seeks to treat the patient in his or her wholeness with the recognition that patient identity includes a person's relationships, religious or spiritual identity and practices, and personal story. Her philosophy of patient care led to the inclusion of social workers, bereavement counselors, chaplains, and volunteers on the hospice caregiving team. A hospice-based anthropology perceives the patient as a socially connected, narrative being with an individual experience of pain. The hospice model of care aligns well with models of narrative medicine that view the clinical encounter as one structured by narrativity. Further, the hospice anthropology offers an approach to patient identity that includes the religious and spiritual dimensions of patient identity and experience, an aspect of personhood that calls for more attention in narrative medicine scholarship. Life review and the conversations that emerge from spiritual assessments function as examples of narrative practices that can occur in the clinical encounter. In the following chapter, I demonstrate the ways in which life review represents a form of moral self-evaluation for patients at the end of life.

NOTES

1. Paul Ricoeur, *Oneself as Another* (Chicago, IL: University of Chicago Press, 1992), 161.
2. Ibid., 162.
3. Ibid., 159–160.
4. Ibid., 318.
5. Ibid., 172.
6. Ricoeur uses the term "solicitude" to speak about his concept of the giving-receiving dialectic at play in ethical relationships on page 188. For his analysis of the limits of Aristotle's and Levinas's ethics, see the seventh and tenth studies of the text.

7. Ricoeur notes in his introduction to *Oneself as Another* that he does not explicitly focus on the religious dimension of human experience in the text. He says that he wants to bracket his own religious views from the philosophical perspective on selfhood that he provides in *Oneself as Another* as well as any need on the part of the reader to assume religious belief for support of his claims. He says, "It will be observed that this asceticism of the argument, which marks, I believe, all my philosophical work, leads to a type of philosophy from which the actual mention of God is absent and in which the question of God, as a philosophical question, itself remains in a suspension that could be called agnostic" (23–24). In dialogue with Ricoeur, Richard Kearney's work builds a bridge between philosophy and theology in which he reimagines a concept of God that creates space for both relationality and uncertainty. See *The God Who May Be: A Hermeneutics of Religion* (Bloomington: Indiana University Press, 2001) and *Anatheism: Returning to God after God* (New York: Columbia University Press, 2010).

8. Cicely M. Saunders, *St. Christopher's in Celebration: Twenty-One Years at Britain's First Modern Hospice* (London: Hodder and Stoughton, 1988).

9. James Lewis Milton, *Medicine and Care of the Dying: A Modern History* (Oxford; New York: Oxford University Press, 2007).

10. Daniel Callahan, *False Hopes: Why America's Quest for Perfect Health Is a Recipe for Failure* (New York: Simon & Schuster, 1998). Though binary, these categories can be helpful as a rhetorical device to analyze distinct medical epistemologies and how patient identity is framed within them.

11. John Cacioppo, professor of psychology at the University of Chicago, developed the field of social neuroscience and researches the effects of loneliness for the elderly. See his book written with William Patrick, *Loneliness: Human Nature and the Need for Social Connection* (New York: W. W. Norton & Co, 2008) as well as the following research on the health consequences of perceived isolation, primarily depression and death: J. T. Cacioppo, M. E. Hughes, L. J. Waite, L. C. Hawkley, and R. A. Thisted, "Loneliness as a Specific Risk Factor for Depressive Symptoms: Cross-Sectional and Longitudinal Analyses," *Psychology and Aging* 21, no. 1 (2006), 140–51, as well as Y. Luo, L. Hawkley, L. Waite, and J. Cacioppo, "Loneliness, Health, and Mortality in Old Age: A National Longitudinal Study," *Social Science & Medicine (1982)* 74, no. 6 (2012): 907–14.

12. Cicely Saunders, "Nature and Management of Terminal Pain," in E. F. Shotter, ed. *Matters of Life and Death* (London: Dartman, Longman, and Todd, 1970), 15–26.

13. Cicely M. Saunders and Mary Baines, *Living with Dying: The Management of Terminal Disease* (Oxford; New York: Oxford University Press, 1983).

14. Ira Byock, *Dying Well: Peace and Possibilities at the End of Life* (New York: Riverhead Books, 1998).

15. Byock notes in *Dying Well* that not all patients prefer to die pain-free. As hospice is structured to honor patient preference, ultimately the decision to receive treatment for pain is left up to the individual patient in dialogue with the hospice care team and medical director.

16. Chi-Keong Ong and Duncan Forbes, "Embracing Cicely Saunders's Concept of Total Pain," *BMJ: British Medical Journal* 331, no. 7516 (2005): 576.

17. Ellen Flaherty, "How to Try This: Using Pain-Rating Scales with Older Adults—This Article Examines Three Pain-Rating Scales—the Numeric Rating Scale, the Verbal Descriptor Scale, and the Faces Pain Scale-Revised—That Are Widely Used with Older Patients," *The American Journal of Nursing* (2008): 40.

18. Caroline Richmond, "Dame Cicely Saunders," *BMJ: British Medical Journal* 331, no. 7510 (2005): 238.

19. Richmond, "Dame Cicely Saunders."

20. NHPCO Fact Sheet, 2012 "Medicare Hospice Conditions of Participation Volunteer 5% Cost Savings Match Information Sheet: A Resource for Volunteer Managers." http://www.nhpco.org/sites/default/files/public/regulatory/Volunteer_Cost_Savings_Information.pdf.

21. "Medicare Hospice Conditions of Participation: Spiritual Caregiver," NHPCO, 5. https://www.nhpco.org/sites/default/files/public/regulatory/Spiritual_tip_sheet.pdf.

22. "Hospice Payment System," Department of Health and Human Services: Centers for Medicare & Medicaid Services," 7. https://www.cms.gov/Outreach-and-Education/Medicare-Learning-Network-MLN/MLNProducts/downloads/hospice_pay_sys_fs.pdf.

23. George Handzo, Kevin Flannelly, et al., "What Do Chaplains Really Do? II. Visitation in the New York Chaplaincy Study," *Journal of Health Care Chaplaincy* 14, no. 1 (2008): 53.

24. C. Mako, K. Galek, and S. Poppito, "Spiritual Pain among Patients with Advanced Cancer in Palliative Care," *Journal of Palliative Medicine* 9 (2006): 1106–1113.

25. Raymond de Vries, Nancy Berlinger, and Wendy Cadge, *Lost in Translation: The Chaplain's Role in Health Care* (The Hastings Center, 2008).

26. Joint Commission, Standards Interpretations FAQs, Medical Record-Spiritual Assessment, found at https://www.jointcommission.org/mobile/standards_information/jcfaqdetails.aspx?StandardsFAQId=1492&StandardsFAQChapterId=31&ProgramId=0&ChapterId=0&IsFeatured=False&IsNew=False&Keyword=.

27. Alexander Tartaglia, "Reflections on the Development and Future of Chaplaincy Education," *Journal of Reflective Practice* 35 (Spring 2015): 116–23. See Wendy Cadge's text *Paging God: Religion in the Halls of Medicine* (Chicago, IL: University of Chicago Press, 2013) for a history of Clinical Pastoral Education and details on the role of chaplaincy in a health-care context.

28. "Hospice Policy Compendium: The Medicare Benefit, Regulations, Quality Reporting, and Public Policy," National Organization of Hospice and Palliative Care, 2016. PDF accessible at https://www.nhpco.org/sites/default/files/public/public_policy/Hospice_Policy_Compendium.pdf.

29. "Medicare Conditions of Participation: Bereavement," NHPCO, https://www.nhpco.org/sites/default/files/public/regulatory/Bereavement_tip_sheet.pdf.

30. The technical definitions of terms related to bereavement care are as follows: bereavement is the "objective situation one faces after having lost an important person via death." Grief is the internal experience in response to the loss; mourning is the outwardly expressed manifestation of the internal experience of grief. From the "Grief, Bereavement, and Loss" PDQ of the Supportive and Palliative Care Editorial

Board. Bethesda, MD: National Cancer Institute, October 8, 2014. https://www.cancer.gov/about-cancer/advanced-cancer/caregivers/planning/bereavement-hp-pdq.

31. 35.5 percent of hospice patients receive services for seven days or less; the median length of care in 2014 was 17.4 days, a consistent figure since 2000. "Hospice Policy Compendium," 11.

32. N. Hooyman and B. Kramer, *Living through Loss; Interventions across the Life Span* (New York; Chichester; West Sussex: Columbia University Press, 2006), 44.

33. From Appendix E: Bereavement Experiences after the Death of a Child, "Children take on great symbolic importance in terms of parents' generativity and hope for the future. All parents have dreams about their children's futures; when a child dies the dreams may die too. This death of future seems integral to the intensity of many parents' responses." Institute of Medicine (US) Committee on Palliative and End-of-Life Care for Children and Their Families; M. J. Field and R. E. Behrman, editors. *When Children Die: Improving Palliative and End-of-Life Care for Children and Their Families* (Washington, DC: National Academies Press, 2003).

34. Paul Bramadat, Harold G. Coward, and Kelli I. Stajduhar, *Spirituality in Hospice Palliative Care* (New York: SUNY Press, 2013), 25.

35. From the Joint Commission's Standards "Frequently Asked Questions." http://www.jointcommission.org/mobile/standards_information/jcfaqdetails.aspx?StandardsFAQId=290&StandardsFAQChapterId=29.

36. From "Introduction to Credentialing," Preceding Standard MS.4.10, Joint Commission on the Accreditation of Health Care Organization, *Comprehensive Accreditation Manual for Hospitals*, 2008.

37. Michael J. Balboni, Christiana M. Puchalski, and John R. Peteet, "The Relationship between Medicine, Spirituality and Religion: Three Models for Integration," *Journal of Religion and Health* 53, no. 5 (2014): 1586.

38. Christina M. Puchalski and David B. Larson, "Developing Curricula in Spirituality and Medicine," *Academic Medicine* 73, no. 9 (1998): 970.

39. Preamble to the Constitution of the World Health Organization as adopted by the International Health Conference, New York, June 19–22, 1946.

40. Also addressed in this article by Farr Curlin and Peter Moschovis, "Is Religious Devotion Relevant to the Doctor-Patient Relationship?" *Journal of Family Practice* 53, no. 8 (2004).

41. Curlin and Moschovis, "Is Religious Devotion Relevant to the Doctor-Patient Relationship?."

42. Daniel P. Sulmasy, *The Rebirth of the Clinic: An Introduction to Spirituality in Health Care* (Washington, DC: Georgetown University Press, 2006).

43. Daniel Sulmasy, "Spirituality, Religion, and Clinical Care," *Chest* 135, no. 6 (2009): 1635.

44. K. M. Trevino, M. Balboni, A. Zollfrank, T. Balboni, and H. G. Prigerson, "Negative Religious Coping as a Correlate of Suicidal Ideation in Patients with Advanced Cancer," *Psycho-Oncology* 23, no. 8 (2014): 936.

45. Daniel Sulmasy, "Spiritual Issues in the Care of Dying Patients: '. . . It's Okay between Me and God,'" *JAMA* 296, no. 11 (2006): 1389.

46. Ibid.

47. Sulmasy, "Spirituality, Religion, and Clinical Care," 1640.

48. Christina Puchalski, "The Role of Spirituality in Health Care." *Proceedings (Baylor University Medical Center)* 14, no. 4 (2001): 352.

49. The requirements for board-certified chaplaincy move beyond introductory or continuing education medical school courses, and the certification process creates a system of accountability, one important in clinical contexts in which patients are often vulnerable and may have limited mobility to leave a scenario that makes them uncomfortable. Ideally, a medical school course on spirituality will emphasize when it is appropriate to offer or request a chaplain referral, rather than promoting the idea that the physician is adequately trained to identify and meet the patient's spiritual or religious needs.

50. C. Puchalski and A. Romer, "Taking a Spiritual History Allows Clinicians to Understand Patients More Fully," *Journal of Palliative Medicine* 3, no. 1. (2000): 129–37.

51. T. Maugans, "The SPIRITual History," *ArchFam Med* 5, no. 1 (1996): 11–16.

52. G. Anandarajah and E. Hight, "Spirituality and Medical Practice: Using the HOPE Questions as a Practical Tool for Spiritual Assessment," *American Family Physician* 63, no. 1 (2001): 81–89.

53. George Fitchett, *Assessing Spiritual Needs: A Guide for Caregivers* (Ohio: Academic Renewal Press, 2002).

54. Gordon W. Allport, *The Individual and His Religion: A Psychological Interpretation* (New York: Macmillan, 1950).

55. Gordon Allport and Michael J. Ross, "Personal Religious Orientation and Prejudice," *Journal of Personality and Social Psychology* 5, no. 4 (Apr 1967): 432–43.

56. One could say that the language of "spirituality" comports with Allport's concept of intrinsic religiosity. However, the very language of religion is anathema to some individuals; many patients identify specifically as spiritual and *not* religious.

57. John Swinton and Richard Payne, *Living Well and Dying Faithfully: Christian Practices for End-of-Life Care* (Grand Rapids, MI: W. B. Eerdmans Pub. Co., 2009).

58. C. Hains and N. J. Hulbert-Williams, "Attitudes toward Euthanasia and Physician-Assisted Suicide: A Study of the Multivariate Effects of Healthcare Training, Patient Characteristics, Religion and Locus of Control," *Journal of Medical Ethics* 39, no. 11 (2013): 713.

59. Bishop, *The Anticipatory Corpse*, 242.

60. Margaret E. Mohrmann, "Ethical Grounding for a Profession of Hospital Chaplaincy," *The Hastings Center Report* 38, no. 6 (2008): 22.

61. Mohrmann, "Ethical Grounding for a Profession of Hospital Chaplaincy."

62. Elaine Scarry, *The Body in Pain: The Making and Unmaking of the World* (New York: Oxford University Press, 1985).

63. Ann Jurecic, *Illness as Narrative* (Pittsburgh: University of Pittsburgh Press, 2012).

Chapter 3

Narrative Ethics and Practices from the Patient's Perspective

Life Review as Ethical Self-Assessment

Questions about ethics and morality for terminal patients often address the right to die or the use of life-prolonging technologies. However, other forms of ethical analysis are present for end-of-life patients that are not by nature dilemma-based. Instead, questions of morality, duty, and appropriate behavior or life in accordance with personal, social, or religious virtues can be present for persons reflecting on the moral arc of their lives. This reflection is often precipitated by an unexpected medical event, and particularly by a terminal diagnosis. Narrative medicine and narrative medical ethics offer a paradigm for understanding this mode of ethical reflection that can occur when patients learn of their prognosis. Narrative medicine centers on the caregiver or clinician and the development of his or her skills in attending a patient, what Charon calls "narrative competence."[1] My concern in this chapter does not have to do with the empathic skills of the clinician, also referred to as the moral imagination of practitioners, in which they learn to consider the experience of the patient they encounter.[2] Rather, because narrative medicine is heavily weighted toward the practitioner, my goal in this chapter is to turn to evaluative process of life review engaged in by the patient particularly as a practice of narrative medicine. A clinician trained in narrative medicine can learn to attend to the narrative practices engaged in by patients such as life review. Because a patient's interior world cannot be fully known, I look to themes that emerge from terminal patients at the end of life both in literature and in reports from clinicians and patients; both offer rich reserves of information for understanding the spectrum of human experience in the face of terminal illness and death.[3] Not all of the patients are engaging in the structured process of life review, though many are engaging in a similar, if informal, process of retrospective reflection and evaluation of their lives. Life review is a common intervention for health care chaplains, and I examine the various modalities of life review that clinicians might encounter or initiate with patients.

Previous research shows that life review has a therapeutic function; here, I suggest that it also has a moral function.[4] In this chapter, I argue that life review in hospice is a form of ethical self-analysis for end-of-life patients who have the necessary verbal and cognitive capacities to do so. The central question being asked in this process of retrospection and self-analysis, either implicitly, or explicitly, is did I live a good life? This question is, fundamentally, an ethics question, though the definition of the good life will differ depending on the person and context. My primary concern is with the process of evaluative retrospection rather than normative claims about what the good life is. It is the patient's attention to his or her individual definition of the good life that interests me in this chapter. Some reach the end of their life with a sense of well-being and satisfaction that they have lived well and are at peace with dying. But for many patients, life review evokes feelings with a negative valence—a sense of incompletion, regret, guilt, and fear, centering on the realization that they did not live their lives as they had hoped and that time is limited for making changes approximating the good life, as they define it.

Hospice is distinct from palliative care in that hospice requires a six-month prognosis if the disease takes its natural course.[5] Palliative care models, which allow both comfort and curative clinical measures, are becoming more common, due to growing clinical education about palliative medicine, the need for programs oriented to chronically ill patients, and because the language of "hospice" continues to unsettle some patients, families, and even clinical caregivers. Because hospice requires a terminal diagnosis and the release of curative care, there is recognition by the patient, the patient's family, and his or her caregivers that death is real and approaching soon. It is because of this honesty about a patient's terminal state that I focus primarily on this population of patients. I claim that a terminal diagnosis and honesty about impending death, combined with a retrospective narrative practice such as life review, creates a situation in which patients turn toward how they lived rather than how they hope to live. It is in this turn toward the past that patients engage in an ethical self-analysis about whether they lived well. While there can be language about how to prepare for a death on the patient's terms and there can be a reframing of what hope means at the end of life, I claim that because one no longer has a future *telos*, engaging in subjunctive understandings of future selfhood, patients then analyze how they in fact did live, according to their recollection and what they value. This ethical self-analysis is influenced by cultural understandings of what it means to fulfill one's social roles and be a good person. Patients are measuring whether or not they lived up to their standards of success.

LIFE REVIEW FOR END-OF-LIFE PATIENTS

R. N. Butler published the first document on structured life review in 1963, four years before the formal establishment of hospice by Cicely Saunders.[6] He claimed that older persons engage in a process of reflection about the course of their lives, particularly as they face life's end. He maintained that this is a universal feature of aging, stating:

> I conceive of the life review as a naturally occurring, universal mental process characterized by the progressive return to consciousness of past experiences, and, particularly, the resurgence of unresolved conflicts; simultaneously, and normally, these revived experiences can be surveyed and reintegrated.[7]

The process of life review is known by other names: reminiscence therapy, retrospection, guided autobiography, and, more recently, storywork.[8] "Dignity therapy" is another term form of life review, specifically designed for end-of-life patients with the goal of achieving closure.[9] For the purpose of clarity, I will primarily use the language of life review to refer to the process of retrospective reflection on the course of one's life, particularly for patients with a terminal diagnosis enrolled in hospice care. Barbara and Barrett Haight use the term "structured life review" building on Butler's idea to create a short-term life review model for both caregivers and clinicians.[10] They attend closely to Erik Erikson's developmental stages of psychosocial development and offer a framework that applies to more than just hospice patients.[11]

Butler believed that a terminal diagnosis can prompt the process of life review; however, one's advanced age alone, or an acute reminder of one's mortality, can similarly lead to this process of reflection on one's life.[12] He describes a person's end of life as being a prime window of time for self-reflection.[13] Recent studies show that there are marked differences in what is considered salient for patients depending on their age and gender. For example, Ando, Morita, and Connor in their study on life review for cancer patients note that the primary concerns for forty-year-olds related to their children, for fifty-year-olds, death, for seventy-year-olds, resignation about their lives, and for eighty-year-olds, relationships with others were their primary concern.[14] Their studies point to the reality that the focus is not merely on an answer to the question, "how did I live?" particularly for younger terminal patients who may be concerned about how to establish a framework of care for their dependent children who will survive them.

There are general themes that are shared for patients engaging in the process of life review, however, Butler made no move to describe life review as one that has an internal structure or order. He did not impose a formula or developmental timeline on the activity, noting that it can involve "stray and seemingly insignificant thoughts about oneself and one's life history."[15] He maintained that the process for some can be inward and solitary, a process in which thoughts happen upon individuals rather than being intentionally called forth.[16] Though Butler conceived of the life review as more of a meandering of thoughts, the process has become formalized in many hospice models. Life is divided into developmental periods connected with one's chronological age. Major historical events are taken into account, shaping how one reflects on the course of one's life.

Though I emphasize the social aspect of life review that the process involves a dialogical interaction often between patient and a nonprofessional visitor or caregiver, for Butler life review can be done individually, even internally in silence.[17] The group process of life review as a shared activity of piecing together and articulating the narrative of one's life is also an option that exists as a way to engage in the process.[18] Butler's primary interest was in what he perceived to be the fact that individuals do engage in this process, rather than the modes in which they do it. In hospice, any attempt to engage in life review would follow attention given to pain and symptom management.[19]

In addition to claiming that life review is a universal activity of reflection, he maintained that life review correlates with advanced age and an awareness of one's mortality. However, the deaths of others, dramatic health or ability changes, and relational or professional disappointments can also trigger a sense that one's life calls for analysis or review. Butler notes that the condemned and that young people with terminal diagnoses engage in this process of reflection; his primary research interest is in the aged population because these are the more ordinary cases, and he felt that there was some neglect of this demographic in clinical research.[20] One of his goals appears to be depathologizing the life review process, noting that it is not an indicator of maledict psychological concern, but an ordinary, and he adds universal, reflective exercise.[21]

Reminiscence versus Life Review

In his article, Butler makes a distinction between reminiscence and life review, defining reminiscence as a process of recollection and life review as a process of evaluation. However, the term "reminiscence" has come to signify what Butler intended to point to when he described life review. Jeffrey Webster prefers the term "reminiscence therapy" or "reminiscence work" to describe the process of evaluating one's life over time. Webster, disagreeing with Butler's claims about the timeline for retrospective reflection, believes that reminiscence occurs throughout a person's lifespan rather than just at the end of life.[22] The primary difference between reminiscence and life review is that reminiscence does not involve the interpretive move.

Language about life review often sounds positive—the process is described in language that connotes feelings of well-being, harmony, justice, and closure. The romantic ideal of the bedside narration of a life well lived comes to mind. However, Butler, a realist about the process based on his experience with it, notes that life review is not necessarily positive and can include experiences of regret, loss, and despair.[23] Haight in her review of the literature following Butler's article notes that almost all the descriptions of the results of life review tend toward the positive.[24] The process of reminiscence is described as healthy, therapeutic, adaptive, and integrative.[25] Haight sees this positive spin as a limitation in the research. Though hospice has an overarching goal of minimizing pain, life review is not necessarily presented as a mode of therapy for patients as a means to address unresolved issues. One could say that the primary form of pain management that life review attends to is the pain that comes from social isolation of the elderly and infirm. Accordingly, there is no need to have the goal of resolving past emotional or relational issues through life review; its purpose is to meet the social needs of patients that can be met through conversation. There is not necessarily a therapeutic goal—that is, "closure"—involved in the process.[26]

Butler described life review as a process of interpretation in which there is a "reorganization of past experiences" that includes recognition and evaluation by the self.[27] This evaluation includes recognition of one's "past inadequacies" that may have gone unexamined if not for the reality of the patient's impending death.[28] To aid in this process, hospice organizations have created guides for retrospection. For instance, the Hospice Foundation of America published "A Guide for Recalling and Telling Your Life Story"; in Europe the Age Concern Society offers "Reminiscence and Recall: A Guide to Good Practice" and "The Reminiscence Trainer's Pack" online to assist those interested in the process.[29]

Ultimately, life review as it functions in hospice is a process of reflection, interpretation, and preparation. Through reflection on the course of one's life, a person engages in the activity of interpreting these experiences according to both internal and external standards.[30] Additionally, life review is a process of preparation for death as one evaluates the time one spent in the world as it stands in the face of the limits of one's time, coming to terms with how one lived. Though life review does not require a terminal diagnosis, or even advanced age, hospice presents an opportunity to engage in the process by explicitly speaking about life review as an activity one can engage in using volunteer services or pastoral care. Also, in hospice, honesty structures the conversation about the time one has left. When one knows time is limited, they may be more inclined to do an assessment of how they lived.

MODALITIES OF LIFE REVIEW

Dignity Therapy

Dignity Therapy, developed by Canadian psychiatrist Harvey Chochinov, is a dialogical model of psychosocial care for terminal patients that focuses primarily on legacy. Chochinov discovered that patients often experienced distress over the recognition that they would no longer exist and would not be remembered by those still living. Dignity Therapy serves as a way to therapeutically address this need by creating a record of the person's narrative as a form of legacy, something that will exist even after they die.[31] Dignity Therapy addresses some of the same questions as life review—questions regarding social roles and matters of pride and acceptance; however, there are two distinct points of difference between the two modalities of narrative medicine. One, life review does not have a purported audience; no one else, aside from the person who serves as facilitator will necessarily hear or read the words of the patient. Two, the approaches have different goals. The goal in Dignity Therapy is to create something to leave behind, something that will live on after the patient has died as a testament to their lives. By design, this would make the narrative established in Dignity Therapy more selective, bringing forward what a patient is most proud of as a signifier of his or her legacy.[32] In contrast, the narrative that emerges in life review is less structured to be positive. Because a person is engaging in self-analysis the result may not be one that the patient is proud of. Rather, the patient may feel deep regret and disappoint due to the realizations that emerge in life review. The very term "Dignity Therapy" can shape the course of conversation; life review, a more neutral term, allows the process to be more patient-directed and open with regard to content. Furthermore, Dignity Therapy is a therapeutic technique, intended to address and mitigate patient distress (the distress that results from the fear of being forgotten). Chochinov reports that in his research on Dignity Therapy, 76 percent of patients reported a heightened sense of dignity following the experience; 68 percent reported feeling an increased sense of purpose in their lives; 67 percent reported a heightened sense of meaning; and 81 percent reported that it had been or would be of help to their family.[33] Overall, 91 percent of participants reported satisfaction with the process. Alternatively, life review in hospice may be less of a therapeutic intervention; in fact, patient distress can increase with the recognition that a patient did not live up to his or her standards combined with the urgency that can attend a terminal diagnosis.

Guided Autobiography

Guided autobiography similarly has a therapeutic function though the purpose includes motives such as striving to "strengthen identity" and to "help older persons come to terms with the lives they have led" which can have a positive or negative valence depending on the person's interpretation.[34] While it is possible that a person's autobiography is one of regret and analysis of moral failings, the guided aspect to the process involves structuring dialogue according to the person doing the guiding. If they believe they "can help older adults build greater understanding and self-worth" in the process, their desire to make the experience positive for the person involved can limit the person's opportunity to do an honest self-analysis, particularly because the narratives written via guided autobiography are shared in a group setting.[35]

Illness Narratives

The term "illness narrative" originated with Arthur Kleinman's text *The Illness Narratives: Suffering, Healing, and the Human Condition* in 1988.[36] Kleinman, both a psychiatrist and an anthropologist, was intrigued by the differences between how illness is interpreted by patients and how it is interpreted by clinicians in the biomedical model of care. Kleinman expands beyond biophysical interpretations of illness to discuss how they shape a person's sense of self and a person's relationships with others. The text was written at approximately the same time as the turn toward narrative in the medical humanities.[37]

Audre Lorde's *The Cancer Journals* is an example of an illness narrative.[38] In this autobiographical account, she writes about how it feels to be unsupported by one's clinical caregivers and it was precisely this feeling of rejection and alienation that motored her to write the text. For Lorde, narration functions as a form of self-healing with the potential to provide healing for others through speaking openly about her experience, in a manner devoid of sentimentality. Lorde's *Cancer Journals* exemplify the genre of autobiography in narrative medicine, with a distinct turn toward narrative medical ethics or how medicine should be performed in her analysis.[39] In this illness narrative, Lorde describes the inner experience—the sense of loss, rage, and abandonment—she feels after her cancer diagnosis and surgery. Lorde uses self-writing and the memoir genre to mourn the changes in her physical body, to recreate her sense of self post-surgery, and to urge other patients, particularly women, to share their individual experiences.[40] By sharing her story, she believes she is removing the veil from what it means to have a "normal" body, that is, a healthy, fully functioning body.

In many illness narratives, Lorde's as an example, one of the author's goals is to express dissatisfaction with care rather than with one's life. Additionally, illness narratives, as the name of the genre expresses, concern how the patient's illness affected or affects his or her life, sense of self, and relationships.[41, 42] In Life Review, the focus is on the patient's life, sense of self, and relationships, but does not necessarily include how the reality of illness informed the patient's interpretation of his or her life. Though some terminal patients have a diagnosis such as cancer or congestive heart failure, this is not the case for all patients. Some are admitted to hospice care with an unspecified diagnosis; they may be dying of advanced age with no categorizable illness to speak of. In these cases, patients do not gain a sense of identity from their illness in the manner that those writing illness narratives do.

Arthur Frank's *The Wounded Storyteller* comes the closest to the concept of the self and the ethical analysis involved in life review. He views the ill person not as a passive recipient of care, but as an agent in how his or her illness is interpreted and shared.[43] It is through the narrative process that the patient reclaims agency. Additional modalities of reminiscence and reflection include videos, memory books, scrapbooks, and communicating via social media; however, these forms of self-narration do not necessarily have the evaluative component that Life Review elicits.[44]

Differences between Other Modalities and Life Review

A primary difference between autobiography and life review is that there is not necessarily a documented or recorded product that comes as a result of the process. Life Review quite simply can involve a patient discussing memories or unrealized plans with a hospice volunteer. There is no established goal beyond the process itself. Similarly, there is no intended audience in life review; however, some chose to document their experiences. In illness narratives and autobiographies, there is an assumed audience; knowing this may inform the content of a patient's narrative. A patient may share his or her regrets and disappoints during the process of life review whereas if a book were being written the negative appraisal one has of one's life may not be discussed. Additionally, life review often occurs with volunteer companions or family members interested in documenting life history. Because the conversation does not occur in a professional context, there is freedom for the patient to speak without worrying about clinical judgment. Ultimately, the process is self-based and the person is his or her own judge of moral behavior.

Capabilities Necessary for Patient Life Review

Forms of life review in hospice include short-term life review and Dignity Therapy.[45] However, unofficial means of life review also exist in the form interview questions based on a person's lived experience. Life review serves multiple purposes: creating a legacy for those who remain, reducing isolation for terminal patients, and reducing depression for patients whose symptoms have reached the limits of pharmacological management. The researchers who developed structured short-term life review maintain that by participating in the dialogical process, patients experience lower psychosocial distress than patients who do not.[46] While not all patients experience a sense of harmony or satisfaction after participating in life review, the process nevertheless can serve as a vehicle for ethical analysis in that it is centered on answering the question, "How did you live?"

Two concepts underlying the process of structured short-term life review in the hospice model of care call for attention. First, the process relies on a linear understanding of time and human development. For instance, the Hospice of Cincinnati suggests an interview format divided into distinct life periods: childhood (birth to thirteen years), adolescence (fourteen to twenty-one years), young adulthood (twenty-two to thirty-two years), middle adulthood (thirty-six to sixty-five years), and older adulthood (sixty-six to ninety-nine years).[47] Scholars such as Galen Strawson challenge the idea that humans share this developmental timeline when reflecting on their lives. Strawson, like Butler, believes memory can be more episodic and fragmented, and that self-narration, for some, centers on an in-the-moment experience of selfhood in time.

Also, the process of life review in the hospice model of care relies on a concept of narrative identity. Telling one's story, reminiscing, pondering one's choices in life, all of these activities require an agency-based understanding of selfhood. Furthermore, a narrative anthropology requires a high level of cognition and lucidity about past and present. Patients who are confused, aphasic, sedated, or in pain may not be able to engage in this process.

LIFE REVIEW IN HOSPICE
AS A MODE OF MORAL REFLECTION

In this section I attempt to demonstrate that life review is not merely a form of reminiscence; rather it is a form of retrospective ethical self-evaluation. There are thematic elements that emerge for patients, disclosing the underlying process of moral reflection and evaluation. Whereas Butler uses the language of "reorganization" of one's understanding of self, I use the language of evaluation.[48] Both terms connote an interpretive move: Butler believes one interprets one's past based on a sense of self one is trying to confirm; I maintain that one evaluates one's past behavior and context based on perceived standards of what it means to be a good person (based on virtues, duty, one's religion, gender, or familial role) as well as standards for the good life, however this is defined by the patient.

Butler maintains that certain patients are more likely to experience depression, anxiety, and despair as a result of life review. Those who have a future orientation, deferring culmination of selfhood to a point of time on the horizon—an "ever receding horizon" to use Karl Rahner's term, are often unsatisfied with the course of their lives.[49] In psychosocial literature, this tendency toward the future, or the fallacy of misplaced meaning, in which one neglects their present circumstances for the promise of future fulfillment shows strong connections with chronic anxiety.[50] The second group of those who have negative responses to life review includes those who have consciously caused harm to others during their lives and they are unable to consider "forgiveness and redemption" as possibilities in their respective futures. Finally, Butler names those who are "arrogant and prideful" as likely to experience distress during life review. Butler extrapolates that "their narcissism is probably particularly disturbed by the realization of death."[51] His claims are speculative, based on his experience as a clinician working with terminal patients. Regarding Butler's third category, Paul Tillich similarly links anxiety and distress about dying with the fear of nonbeing in his text *The Courage to Be*.[52]

Butler repeatedly points to the image of the mirror and the activity of "mirror-gazing" as relevant to his description of life review. What calls for attention is not necessarily that the person is looking in the mirror, but that they do not recognize who they see. They see a stranger before them—the reflection does not depict the person they desire to see. Mirror-gazing prompts the questioning of identity and satisfaction with one's sense of self that parallels the moral evaluation that occurs in life review.[53] A patient realizes that at the culmination of life, when there is no time left for future development of self, one's life was not fully lived. As Milton Lewis notes in his research on the retrospective turn, "life review, by its very nature, evokes a sense of regret and sadness at the brevity of life, the missed opportunities, the mistakes, the wrongs done to others, the chosen paths that turned out badly."[54] In addition to the moral analysis that occurs, distressing realizations emerge that can increase patient suffering at the end of life: fear of loss of self, of being a burden, loss of independence, and loneliness are reported by some patients.[55]

Not all patients engaging in life review experience regret or disappointment in how their lives took shape. Reports of regret signify the gap between how patients interpret how they lived and how patients believe they ought to have lived, pointing to an ethical analysis at work. However, satisfaction with one's life also points to an ethical analysis: a patient did in fact achieve his or her "good life." Others may have a nostalgic version of the past, one in which they romanticize their behavior and possibly long for a false utopia. Butler addresses this tendency when he speaks about the construct of the "fantasy" of the past as utopian, pointing to this interpretation as an example of how one retrospectively organizes his or her sense of self.[56]

Even when a patient experiences a negative appraisal of self, there can be identity formation at the end of life. Both Butler and Erik Erikson maintain that human development does not end in adulthood—that ultimately it has no finish line, apart from death. Hospice clinicians, volunteers, and bereaved family members similarly note that personal change can occur even within a short time frame with the specter of death precipitating life review and attempts at reconciliation.[57]

To make the religious turn in ethical self-analysis, when there is no concept of God in one's moral or religious framework, this activity of weighing good and bad behavior shifts to the person. For those who believe in a judging God (Christians and Muslims, in particular) the self-judgment may feel preemptive; in such evaluative paradigms, it is up to God to decide at death how one lived one's life. However, patients can nevertheless anticipate God's judgement based on their own interpretation of their moral failings.[58]

THEMES THAT POINT TO ETHICAL ANALYSIS

There are multiple themes that emerge in life review, in both formally structured life review and in informal moments of reminiscence and retrospective reflection that point to a process of ethical self-analysis. Through life review, one analyzes, interprets, and both celebrates and grieves one's choices in life. I categorize the themes that follow into two categories, an agency analysis and a context analysis. Agency refers to choices on the part of the patient in which they exercise the most control. Context refers to the patient's experience that they did not choose (family of origin, location of birth and dependent care, etc.). Both of these categories show an ethical analysis at work; the latter primarily using language of justice or fairness. There are three types of speech for end-of-life patients that point to this process of ethical self-evaluation: regret over choices and missed opportunities, the desire for forgiveness, and grief over lost time/longing for more time.

Regret

Because hospice requires a terminal diagnosis, honesty structures conversation about one's prognosis. Awareness about impending death means that when patients are reflecting on ethical questions they turn their awareness to the past. Instead of asking, "How should I live?" a patient instead will turn the question to the past asking, "How did I live?" Life review thus becomes an on-the-ground form of ethical self-evaluation. Patients can reflect on their individual choices, inquiring as to whether they lived up to their own particular expectations. These expectations are influenced by social roles: was I a good mother? did I do the job I wanted to do? The person is engaging in a role-based form of retrospective self-analysis, one shaped by social norms. As Daniel Sulmasy notes drawing from Aristotle's poetics, every ethos requires a mythos.[59] In other words, character development requires a plot. Life review addresses both how one interprets one's character in an agency-based analysis as well as how one interprets one's context in an environmental analysis. One study on regret shows that there are two forms of regret: regret over one's choices and regret over one's "hard times" or the conditions one had no control over. For example, women experiencing regret related to their context report wishing they had had the opportunity to pursue their educations but were unable to do so because of external limitations.[60]

The feeling of regret for terminal patients demonstrates ethical self-analysis. In nurse Bonnie Ware's observation on the top five regrets of the dying, one of the primary regrets is not living one's authentic life—living the "good life" according to social expectations rather than living one's own good life.[61] Because time narrows for terminal patients, pointing them to their final *telos*, the reality that they no longer have behavioral choices in front of them is brought into sharp relief. The limits of autonomy related to action become starkly apparent. Choices related to how one interprets one's life exist, but ultimately one does not have the option of living a different life. Regret and self-reproach point to this recognition. For Ivan Ilyich, for instance, his suffering is compounded by his interpretation that he did not live the right life for him. His pain is more than just physical, a concept of pain that Cicely Saunders recognized in her formulation of "total pain." In fact, after he comes to the conclusion that his life was a lie, he can no longer speak coherently and only screams in pain.[62]

A scene from *The Death of Ivan Ilyich* captures this sense of regret and confusion, a time when one considers the possibility that perhaps the life one lived was not the best life:

> There was something good for me as a child, but that person is no more. Then in law school there was something genuinely good there—enjoyment, friendship, hopes. There were good moments in my Governor's service, and I remember love for women. As I think through my life, there is less and less good. My marriage—at first so happy, then disillusion. The hypocrisy, the anxieties about money all those twenty years.
>
> So what is this? What is it for? Surely it can't be that my life was so pointless, so wrong? And if it was that wrong and that pointless, then why die and die in pain? Something's not right here. Maybe I didn't live as I should. But how could that be, when I did everything I should have done?[63]

Ivan is in extreme physical pain; however, his distress is not limited to his physical experience. As the doctor notes, "his physical suffering is intense, but his spiritual suffering is worse, and that is what torments him most of all."[64]

Cicely Saunders categorizes feelings of regret under spiritual pain, noting that because of growing secularity in the western world, few patients will use explicitly religious language to describe their pain.[65] One could say that the desire to confess points to a form of spiritual pain; however, I am using the language of regret instead to demonstrate that one recognizes that one failed to live up to an assumed standard and that the individual becomes the judge of moral standing rather than a divine being. Saunders also includes a feeling of meaninglessness in her concept of spiritual pain.[66] Instead, a feeling of meaninglessness could come from a nonreligious awareness that one's life did not serve any larger purpose beyond the self. This distress, then, is the result of a form of secular moral analysis rather than being a manifestation of spiritual pain in the way that Saunders sees it. When a patient maintains that his or her life had no meaning or was worthless, a normative ideal underlies this claim. This evaluation presumes that there *should* be a purpose to one's life that transcends self-gratification. A patient is reflecting on the gap between how one lived and how one thinks one ought to have lived.[67]

Desire for Forgiveness

One action that speaks to the process of moral self-reflection for end-of-life patients is that of asking for forgiveness.[68] While expressions of love and gratitude are also noted for end-of-life patients, these have less to do with a moral self-analysis. The desire for forgiveness on the part of patients shows that there is recognition of behavior in which a patient did not live up to his or her expectations. In some patients, unexpressed requests for forgiveness (to receive or be offered forgiveness) correlate with depression.[69]

Patient requests for forgiveness demonstrate this ethical analysis at play. Episodic depression can also be linked to the awareness that one did not live up to one's expectations. There is no universal "standard" here for a good life, there is only the claim that the patient has a standard combined with the recognition that this standard is shaped by moral norms. For example, a person may not have the "burden" of high expectations in life and may not feel the gap between who they aspired to be and who they are. One could even say that this sense of dissatisfaction of not being good enough is either a luxury or a sign of moral self-centeredness. As Ira Byock says, "you die how you live" and a chronic sense of inadequacy that a patient feels in life may also be present at death.[70]

Requests for forgiveness, while they historically may have been categorized as belonging in the spiritual domain, point to an ethical self-analysis rather than exclusively a religious analysis. It has been argued that whereas before the minister was seen as the arbiter of moral concerns, this position transitioned to the doctor (as judge of whether one "lived well") or to the self.[71]

Grief over Lost Time

There can be existential distress when a patient faces a terminal diagnosis. However, this distress can involve more than just an awareness that one will die. One can also mourn the time they had but that they did not use well, grieving missed opportunities, relationships, or a sense of fullness of life. The question, then, is not how can I die well or have a good death, but rather, did I live well? Did I have a good life?[72]

To return to the scenario in *The Death of Ivan Ilyich*, when faced with death Ivan begins to question how he lived his life:

> What if in reality the whole of my life was not done right? Could it be true that I have lived my whole life not as I should have done? It occurs to me that I never did fight against what people in high positions deemed good when they were wrong . . . I shrugged it off. And my work and the construction of my life and my family and my social and professional interest—all of them might not be the right thing. And if this is so, and I am leaving life in the knowledge that I have ruined everything that was given to me and it can't be put right, then what? All of my life was not the right thing, all of it was a dreadful, vast lie.[73]

In this form of analysis, patients evaluate how they lived their lives. There is no set standard for this analysis, no normative framework for "the good life." While no set standard exists, this does not mean that this process does not occur, a process adapted to the individual and one with various manifestations. If one asks oneself, "Did I live well according to my circumstances?" the circumstances will inevitably vary. Also, I do not mean to say that a person will explicitly ask oneself this question and then process his or her response externally, only that a form of ethical analysis occurs if the patient has the necessary cognitive ability to engage in the process.

A consequence of ethical self-analysis is a sense of deep grief over how one lived one's life or a sense of a longing for more time so that one can live one's authentic life. Augustine's *Confessions*, for example, is a narrative of his grief over lost time with God. One can hear his longing in his words of lament, "Late have I loved you, Beauty, so ancient and so new."[74] With regard to the experience of grief, I am not including depression in this category, because, though depression often manifests for terminal patients there are confounding variables for this condition.[75] Depression can result from limited mobility, isolation, sleep deprivation, and other physical factors unrelated to the process of ethical self-evaluation of life review. My overall claim that life review is a process of moral self-reflection corresponds with Cicely Saunder's recognition of the social and spiritual pain patients can feel at the end of life. I suggest that life review, though often presented as therapeutic or sweetly nostalgic, can unearth sources of pain for patients who reflect on their lives, and can be a source of pain itself.

LIFE REVIEW AND THE LIMITS OF RICOEUR'S CONCEPT OF "LIFE PLAN"

Ricoeur uses the language of "life plan" to describe his understanding of agency. Ricoeur's interest is in how the ethical self is understood in ways as a projection toward the future. He speaks of the ethical "aim" for instance, in his petit ethics, aiming for the good life, with and for others in just institutions. In hospice this future orientation can be present, for instance, one can desire to repair relationships, go on trip, or plan one's funeral or last wishes for care. However, I suggested earlier in this chapter that a terminal diagnosis often compels a person to look backward rather than forward, analyzing how one did live instead of how one plans to live in the future. When one makes the retrospective turn, the relevance of "aim" speak diminishes; the future self, the agent of Ricoeur's "life plan" becomes less compelling. One's historical life, embellished by memory or fiction as it may be, exists then as more content-based, more fixed in time, than one's idea of a future self. One then makes the backward turn and analyzes how one lived according to a moral framework.

This analysis, however, does not require a life plan. It requires only the recognition that one did not live the way one could have lived or ought to have lived. Ricoeur's "I can" understanding of agency reaches its earthly limit and one realizes that there was lost time or opportunity in one's life, regardless of whether or not these opportunities were a part of someone's life plan or plot. That is to say, one can engage in this form of ethical self-analysis without comparing how one lived to a fixed ideal of how one hoped to live according to an established life plan. One can consider the course of one's life and feel deep satisfaction that one did in fact live an authentic life (this model does not have to be achievement-based). Reflecting on the question, "How did I live?" is distinct from reflecting on the question, "Did I achieve my life plan?" Also, it is debatable whether or not one even has a "life plan"; for some limited by trauma, they can experience a sense of fore-shortened future, having no expectation of a projected self. Others, as Galen Strawson argued, have a more episodic concept of self in time.[76]

For Ricoeur, the "I can" concept of capability has four parts: I can speak, I can act, I can recount, and I can impute (and be imputed).[77] For those able to recount, they can interpret their lives according to how they spoke, acted, and were responsible. For those terminal patients who cannot speak or cannot recount their lives, it is the interpretation of others that contributes to their identity. When applying Ricoeur's understanding of agency to the process of life review as it exists in the hospice philosophy of care, it becomes clear that the ability to recount is an important one. To expand on Ricoeur, a patient engaging in life review will use their ability to recount their story, naming and analyzing the ways in which one spoke and acted (shifting the "I can" understandings of "I can speak" and "I can act" to the past tense, thus reflecting on how one spoke and acted). The first three capabilities Ricoeur names—speaking, acting, and recounting—function as key features in life review. For patients challenged by cognitive and verbal limits, the ability to speak, act, and recount contracts or disappears entirely. However, Ricoeur's modalities of narrative selfhood continue to be relevant, particularly when looking at the activity of recounting and the activity of imputation.

The activity of recounting continues to hold value for concepts of narrative selfhood for end-of-life patients because this activity does not have to be engaged in by the person involved. A patient's family members, friends, and colleagues, even neighbors or professional caregivers can narrate the person's life and work to create narrative identity on the person's behalf. This is not to say that a witness's testimony is accurate, only that the activity of recounting as it relates to narrative identity remains possible for patients who are unable to narrate their lives themselves. Though there may be some epistemic distance between the life of the patient and the observer describing the life of the patient, this distance does not call for rejecting the observer's perspective. Furthermore, the accuracy of a person's first-person narrative is also questionable, particularly in medicine.[78] The clinical encounter is by nature goal-based, though the goals of the patient and the goals of the clinician may differ, and because the encounter is goal-based, information is selected to represent and support one's goal. By goal, I do not mean "agenda" such as a treatment agenda on the part of the clinician or drug-seeking behavior on the part of a patient; rather, in an admittedly general sense, the goal of the clinician is a diagnosis followed by a plan of care, and the goal of the patient is to receive care and make sense of the events occurring to the body or mind.

This is all to say that narrative identity continues to be possible for end-of-life patients who are themselves unable to offer an account of their lives. These accounts can be offered vicariously and work to establish a narrative identity for patients. In ways, the analysis offered by witnesses can be perceived as more substantial than the one provided by the patient. If the question for analysis is what kind of parent was the patient—the best person to answer this question may be the child, not the parent. Ricoeur noted this situation in his fourth capability, that of imputation. Imputation is a category of narrative identity that creates space for accusing and being accused. Ricoeur includes misconduct, neglect, even malevolence into the category of imputation, recognizing that identity includes brokenness and the possibility of evil.[79]

Narrative identities constructed by those who speak on behalf of the patient also point to the social aspect of Ricoeur's understanding of selfhood: that all identity is mediated, both by ourselves and by others. Identity is filtered through memory, interpretations provided by others, and through a conflation of one's sense of self with the characters that exist in our imagination, characters that we encounter through fiction that we relate to on a deep level. When it comes to applying Ricoeur's concept of selfhood to compromised patients, there are some gaps, however. The places where Ricoeur's concept of narrative identity reach their limits are cases in which patients appear to lack self-awareness or self-recognition (the term "self-esteem" is used in *Oneself as Another*, but that connotes a positivity that does not accurately portray Ricoeur's view of identity). Though the question, "Who am I?" captivates Ricoeur, this question assumes a level of cognitive ability that does not exist for all patients. While self-recognition may not be possible for such patients, there is still value in Ricoeur's concept of attestation when it comes to understanding narrative identity through relationality, even for patients who are unable to offer a coherent narrative themselves.

Ricoeur's concept of the self holds value for analyzing the process of life review and for how to approach the epistemic value of the narrative accounts provided in the process because he recognizes that memory involves a fictional component—that our stories can never be pure fact, just as fictional narratives rely on a truth-base and are not complete inventions of the author. The issue at hand is not whether the patient's claims represent a "true" biography; facticity is not the concern. The concern, rather, is with the value of the process for the patient, with the additional value of possibly having a first-person record of an ordinary person's life that would be lost with the person's death. The person's memories, therefore, do not necessarily have to be true to be valuable because the standard of evaluation is not the one based on external verification. Ultimately, it is the process of reflection and ethical evaluation that is valuable, rather than the veracity of the patient's claims.

CONCLUSION

Life review is a narrative practice of moral self-assessment individuals can engage in following a health crisis or when facing a terminal diagnosis. In this dialogical exchange between patients and caregivers, a patient examines and interprets decisions and actions made during life drawing on the patient's moral framework and, if applicable, religious ethics. Expressions of regret, the desire for forgiveness, and grief over lost time point to the ethical dimensions of life review and are manifestations of moral self-judgement, an individual's reflection on classic ethics questions—what is the good life? Did I live well? The practice of life review serves as a common intervention for health care chaplains trained to meet with patient's as they process their existential distress. Narrative medicine provides a method to prepare for the deep listening involved in life review with patients. Paul Ricoeur's view of identity as narratival, social, and embodied offers an approach to understanding patient identity that aligns well with practices in narrative medicine such as life review.

NOTES

1. Rita Charon, *Narrative Medicine: Honoring the Stories of Illness* (Oxford: Oxford University Press, 2008).

2. John D. Engel, *Narrative in Health Care: Healing Patients, Practitioners, Profession, and Community* (Oxford; New York: Radcliffe Publishing, 2008).

3. The play *W;t* by Margaret Edson (New York: Faber & Faber, 1999) is just one example of the value of literature and dramatic works for considering the experience of terminal patients, even if fictional. Because the scholars I look to do not necessarily use interview or other qualitative forms of data collection, I do not describe the research I draw on as exclusively ethnographic. However, for detailed ethnographic research on illness narratives, see the scholarship of Byron Good, *Medicine, Rationality, and Experience: An Anthropological Perspective* (Cambridge; New York: Cambridge University Press, 1994). See also the work of Mary-Jo DelVecchio Good, *Pain as Human Experience: An Anthropological Perspective* (Berkeley: University of California Press, 1992).

4. Barbara K. Haight and Barrett S. Haight, *The Handbook of Structured Life Review* (Baltimore: Health Professions Press, 2007). Previous research also shows the value of the process: Barbara K. Haight, "The Therapeutic Role of a Structured Life Review Process in Homebound Elderly Subjects," *Journal of Gerontology* 43, no. 2 (1988), 40; B. Mastel-Smith, B. Binder, A. Malecha, G. Hersch, L. Symes and J. McFarlane, "Testing Therapeutic Life Review Offered by Home Care Workers to Decrease Depression among Home-Dwelling Older Women," *Issues in Mental Health Nursing* 27, no. 10 (2006): 1037.

5. Diane E. Meier, "Palliative Care in Hospitals," *JHM Journal of Hospital Medicine* 1, no. 1 (2006): 21.

6. Robert Butler, "The Life Review: An Interpretation of Reminiscence in the Aged," *Psychiatry* 26 (1963): 65. Sharan Merriam questions the universal nature of Butler's claim and the connection he makes between death awareness and life review. See "Butler's Life Review: How Universal Is It?" in *The Meaning of Reminiscence and Life Review*, ed. Jon Hendricks (Amityville, NY: Baywood Pub. Co., 1995).

7. Robert Butler, *The Life Review: An Interpretation of Reminiscence in the Aged*, 65–76.

8. James E. Birren, Donna E. Deutchman, *Guiding Autobiography Groups for Older Adults: Exploring the Fabric of Life* (Baltimore: Johns Hopkins University Press, 1991); William Randall, "Storywork: Autobiographical Learning in Later Life," *ACE New Directions for Adult and Continuing Education* 2010, no. 126 (2010): 25.

9. Harvey Max Chochinov, *Dignity Therapy: Final Words for Final Days* (Oxford; New York: Oxford University Press, 2012). The question of "achievement" is on that calls for analysis, particularly if vulnerable patients feel compelled to seek closure to satisfy his or her clinicians when this is not a goal or event that interests the patient.

10. Haight and Haight, *The Handbook of Structured Life Review*.

11. Erik H. Erikson, *The Life Cycle Completed: Extended Version with New Chapters on the Ninth Stage of Development by Joan M. Erikson* (New York: W. W. Norton, 1998). Haight and Haight, and others building on Erikson's developmental framework of selfhood, look to his stage "Integrity versus Despair" for concepts of identity in the elderly.

12. Butler, *The Life Review: An Interpretation of Reminiscence in the Aged*, 67.

13. M. Lewis and R. Butler, "Life-Review Therapy: Putting Memories to Work in Individual and Group Psychotherapy," *Geriatrics* 29, no. 11 (1974): 165.

14. M. Ando, T. Morita, S. O'Connor, "Primary Concerns of Advanced Cancer Patients Identified through the Structured Life Review Process: A Qualitative Study Using a Text Mining Technique," *Palliative & Supportive Care* 5, no. 3 (2007): 265.

15. Butler, *The Life Review*, 68.

16. Ibid., 65.

17. Ibid., 67.

18. James E. Birren and Kathryn N. Cochran, *Telling the Stories of Life through Guided Autobiography Groups* (Baltimore: Johns Hopkins University Press, 2001).

19. Robert A. Neimeyer, *Techniques of Grief Therapy: Creative Practices for Counseling the Bereaved* (New York: Routledge, 2012).

20. Butler, *The Life Review: An Interpretation of Reminiscence in the Aged*, 65–67.

21. Ibid., 65. He notes, "The prevailing tendency is to identify reminiscence in the aged with psychological dysfunction and thus to regard it essentially as a symptom." His research strives to normalize the process of life review. David Haber describes him as successful in his work to minimize the stigma against reminiscence in the elderly. See David Haber, "Life Review: Implementation, Theory, Research, and

Therapy," *International Journal of Aging and Human Development* 63, no. 2 (2006): 153.

22. Jeffrey Dean Webster and Mary E. Mccall, "Reminiscence Functions across Adulthood: A Replication and Extension," *Journal of Adult Development* 6, no. 1 (1999): 73.

23. James E. Birren, *Encyclopedia of Gerontology* (Amsterdam; Boston: Academic Press, 2007).

24. Hendricks, *The Meaning of Reminiscence and Life Review*.

25. Ibid., 25

26. Describing the popular concept as a myth, Nancy Burns disputes the very existence of closure in her book, *Closure: The Rush to End Grief and What It Costs Us* (Philadelphia, PA: Temple University Press, 2011). To address closure from an ethics perspective, one could say it stems from a well-meaning, but paternalistic, desire for the clinician to facilitate justice or harmony for a patient in distress.

27. Butler, *The Life Review: An Interpretation of Reminiscence in the Aged*, 65–76. He uses the language of the ego to talk about the self's perspective, 68.

28. Ibid., 66.

29. *A Guide for Recalling and Telling Your Life Story* (Washington, DC: Hospice Foundation of America, 2001); Gibson, F., *Reminiscence and Recall: Second Edition* (United Kingdom: Age Concern, 1998); Gibson, F., *Reminiscence Trainer's Pack* (United Kingdom: Age Concern, 2000). Robert Butler offers a succinct overview of life review in. "Age, Death, and Life Review," in *Living with Grief: Loss in Later Life*, ed. Doka, Kenneth J., John Breaux, and Jack D. Gordon (Washington, DC: Hospice Foundation of America, 2002).

30. Hilde Lindemann, *Damaged Identities, Narrative Repair* (Ithaca, NY: Cornell University Press, 2001).

31. Chochinov, *Dignity Therapy: Final Words for Final Days*.

32. Ibid. Interview questions include, "What about yourself or your life are you most proud of?" and "How do you want to be remembered?" See table 2.1 on page 39. These questions structure the type of responses that follow, skewing to the positive. Chochinov does note that for some individuals their "legacy" is that their lives serve as a warning to others, a cautionary tale about how not to live.

33. H. Chochinov, T. Hack, T. Hassard, L. Kristjanson, S. McClement, and M. Harlos, "Dignity Therapy: A Novel Psychotherapeutic Intervention for Patients Near the End of Life," *Journal of Clinical Oncology: Official Journal of the American Society of Clinical Oncology* 23, no. 24 (2005): 5520.

34. James E. Birren, Donna E. Deutchman, *Guiding Autobiography Groups for Older Adults: Exploring the Fabric of Life* (Johns Hopkins University Press, 1991), x.

35. James E. Birren and Kathryn N. Cochran, *Telling the Stories of Life through Guided Autobiography Groups* (Baltimore, MD: Johns Hopkins University Press, 2001), 1.

36. Arthur Kleinman, *The Illness Narratives: Suffering, Healing, and the Human Condition* (New York: Basic Books, 1988).

37. Ann Jurecic, *Illness as Narrative* (Pittsburgh, PA: University of Pittsburgh Press, 2012). Jurecic credits the AIDS epidemic and the campaign to reshape social understandings of the disease as the signpost for when illness narratives emerged as a genre.

38. Audre Lorde, *The Cancer Journals* (San Francisco: Aunt Lute Books, 1997).
39. Lorde, *Cancer Journals*.
40. Ibid., 24–25.
41. Jurecic, in *Illness as Narrative*, attends to the content of illness narratives, noting neglect of critical attention to the genre by literary critics who may feel the need to treat illness narratives with care rather than critical analysis or who, alternatively, view illness narratives as motivated to elicit sympathy rather than literary criticism.
42. Talcott Parsons, "The Sick Role and the Role of the Physician Reconsidered," *The Milbank Memorial Fund Quarterly.Health and Society* 53, no. 3 (1975): 257. In this article he emphasizes that, though the patient and doctor are in an asymmetrical relationship, the patient is not passive in the role as "sick person."
43. Arthur W. Frank, *The Wounded Storyteller: Body, Illness, and Ethics* (Chicago: University of Chicago Press, 1995).
44. M. Lewis, "Life-Review Therapy: Putting Memories to Work in Individual and Group Psychotherapy," *Geriatrics* 29, no. 11 (1974): 165–73.
45. Ando Michiyo, et al., "Efficacy of Short-Term Life-Review Interviews on the Spiritual Well-being of Terminally Ill Cancer Patients," *Journal of Pain and Symptom Management* 39, no. 6 (2010): 993.
46. Michiyo, et al., "Efficacy of Short-Term Life-Review Interviews on the Spiritual Well-Being of Terminally Ill Cancer Patients," 993.
47. Hospice of Cincinnati, http://www.hospiceofcincinnati.org/life_review_info.shtml.
48. Butler, *The Life Review: An Interpretation of Reminiscence in the Aged*, 69.
49. Ibid., 70. Karl Rahner, *Foundations of Christian Faith: An Introduction to the Idea of Christianity* (New York: Seabury Press, 1978).
50. David H. Barlow, "Unraveling the Mysteries of Anxiety and Its Disorders from the Perspective of Emotion Theory," *American Psychologist American Psychologist* 55, no. 11 (2000): 1247.
51. Butler, *The Life Review: An Interpretation of Reminiscence in the Aged*, 65–76.
52. Paul Tillich, *The Courage to Be* (New Haven, CT: Yale University Press, 1952).
53. Butler, *The Life Review: An Interpretation of Reminiscence in the Aged*, 68, 75.
54. Lewis, "Life-Review Therapy," 165–73.
55. M. Dees, M. Vernooij-Dassen, W. Dekkers, K. Vissers, and C. van Weel, "'Unbearable Suffering': A Qualitative Study on the Perspectives of Patients Who Request Assistance in Dying," *Journal of Medical Ethics* 37, no. 12 (2011): 727.
56. Butler, *The Life Review: An Interpretation of Reminiscence in the Aged*, 65–76.
57. Susan C. Miller, Pedro Gozalo, and Vincent Mor, "Hospice Enrollment and Hospitalization of Dying Nursing Home Patients," *The American Journal of Medicine* 111, no. 1 (2001): 38. In this article the authors address the challenges of late referrals, particularly with regard to the limits posed on psychosocial and spiritual care for the patient.

58. Butler, *The Life Review: An Interpretation of Reminiscence in the Aged*, 65–76. Butler has a patient that uses this language.

59. Daniel P. Sulmasy, "Ethos, Mythos, and Thanatos: Spirituality and Ethics at the End of Life," *Journal of Pain and Symptom Management* 46, no. 3 (2013): 447. Sulmasy expands on Aristotle's poetics to include religion in the category of mythos.

60. E. Timmer, G. Westerhof, F. Dittmann-Kohli, "'When Looking Back on My Past Life I Regret . . .': Retrospective Regret in the Second Half of Life," *Death Studies* 29, no. 7 (2005): 625.

61. Bonnie Ware, *Top Five Regrets of the Dying* (Hay House, Inc., 2012).

62. Leo Tolstoy and Lynn Solotaroff, *The Death of Ivan Illyich* (Toronto; New York: Bantam Books, 1985).

63. Tolstoy and Solotaroff, *The Death of Ivan Illyich*.

64. Engel, *Narrative in Health Care: Healing Patients, Practitioners, Profession, and Community.*

65. Saunders and Baines, *Living with Dying*, 62.

66. Ibid., 63.

67. It calls for attention here that not all persons believe their lives have value and therefore may not even have the luxury of expecting to think that their lives should "serve a purpose." The expectation that one should have a basic level of self-esteem is one that points to the assumption that all lives are recognized outwardly and inwardly as valuable.

68. Betty Ferrell et al., "Nurses' Responses to Requests for Forgiveness at the End of Life," *Journal of Pain and Symptom Management* 47, no. 3 (2014).

69. J. Exline et al., "Forgiveness, Depressive Symptoms, and Communication at the End of Life: A Study with Family Members of Hospice Patients," *Journal of Palliative Medicine* 15, no. 10 (2012).

70. Ira Byock, *Dying Well: Peace and Possibilities at the End of Life* (Riverhead Books: 1998).

71. M. Therese Lysaught, *On Moral Medicine: Theological Perspectives in Medical Ethics.* (Grand Rapids, MI: W. B. Eerdmans Pub. Co., 2012), 12–21. Cited from Roy Branson's article "The Secularization of American Medicine" originally published in *The Hastings Center Studies* 1, no. 2 (1973): 17–28.

72. My research attends to terminal adults; in the case of pediatric hospice care, parents may grieve over the loss of their child's potential life. The research of Ken Doka and Therese Rando offers nuanced scholarship on grief and mourning as it relates to the loss of a child. For instance, for parental loss of a child see the following representative example by Therese Rando, "An Investigation of Grief and Adaptation in Parents Whose Children Have Died from Cancer," *Journal of Pediatric Psychology* 8, no. 1 (1983): 3.

73. Engel, *Narrative in Health Care: Healing Patients, Practitioners, Profession, and Community*, 161.

74. Gibb Augustine, *The Confessions of Augustine* (New York: Garland Pub., 1980).

75. B. Mastel-Smith et al., *Testing Therapeutic Life Review Offered by Home Care Workers to Decrease Depression among Home-Dwelling Older Women*, 1037–49.

76. Galen Strawson, "Against Narrativity," *Ratio* 17, no. 4 (2004b): 428.

77. Paul Ricoeur, *Memory, History, Forgetting* (Chicago: University of Chicago Press, 2004).

78. Kathryn Montgomery, *Doctors' Stories: The Narrative Structure of Medical Knowledge* (Princeton, NJ: Princeton University Press, 1991), 62.

79. Ricoeur's concept of the misuse of freedom and its attendant guilt that he speaks to in both Paul Ricoeur, *Fallible Man* (New York: Fordham University Press, 1986); Paul Ricoeur, *The Symbolism of Evil* (New York: Harper & Row, 1967). Butler notes that such individuals have a particularly challenging time when evaluating their lives (Butler, *The Life Review*, 70).

Chapter 4

The Limits of Narrative Medicine for End-of-Life Patients

In the previous chapter, I examined life review as a mode of moral analysis for end-of-life patients, particularly for those enrolled in hospice care. My claim was that patients facing the end of their lives often engage in a form of ethical analysis, a narrative process of self-analysis in which they assess their choices, contexts, roles, and limits in life retrospectively. Moral assessments incorporate culturally informed categories—gender, marital status, family role, religious involvement, major life events, and other culturally informed identity markers that vary depending on how the person interprets his or her experience, context, and life events. The process is reconstructive, selective, and idiosyncratic. Themes emerge that demonstrate a preoccupation with judgment. Behaviors at the end of life such as requests for forgiveness, an expressed longing for more time, and regret over missed opportunities or past behaviors point to the function of moral evaluation for end-of-life patients. The desire for confession and a fear of divine judgment or punishment points to the religious dimension of retrospective life review. Though the content of analysis may vary from person to person, especially taking into account demographics and social context, the process nevertheless discloses a form of ethical self-evaluation.

In this chapter, I examine the limits of narrative methods for end-of-life patients who have dementia.[1] While the merits of life review hold true for patients able and interested in the process, there are situations in which the process is compromised for certain populations of patients, particularly patients already marginalized due to their physical and cognitive states. In this chapter I identify these limits, noting the ways the process of life review can be expanded beyond verbal or strictly narrative methods.

LIMITATIONS TO PATIENT'S ABILITIES:
Cognitive Decline and the Impaired Ability to Narrate Coherently

As life expectancy continues to increase in the United States, so does the likelihood of experiencing some form of cognitive decline as one ages.[2] Life review remains possible even with slowed or altered mentation; however, there are forms of cognitive impairment that significantly impede a person's ability to engage in the type of coherent verbal narration expected in encounters structured by the goals of narrative medicine. Alzheimer's disease, the most common form of dementia representing 60 to 80 percent of those affected, impairs cognition over time, compromising a patient's memory and ability to think and speak coherently.[3] The disease leads to death, with progression of the disease often extending over many years.[4] Decline in cognitive and motor function is inevitable; however, the disease progresses differently and manifests distinct symptomology depending on the patient. A patient may demonstrate disorientation and confusion regarding time, believing that he or she is experiencing a period in the past, yet be able to describe this experience with clarity. The content of the account does not align with reality; however, the structure of the account is coherent. In some cases there is a blend of reality and a constructed reality. When a patient describes an event that occurred, but embellishes or confuses the content of the account, details concerning location, subject matter, and the players involved, a type of speech called "confabulation" exists.[5] Confabulation describes an account that is partly true and partly constructed, recognized as such by the listener. The person speaking in a confabulated manner typically defends the validity of the account, possibly to protect a threatened sense of identity. As cognitive and verbal ability declines with the progression of the disease, awareness of one's environment and the ability to attune to conversation with others becomes impaired. Whereas in the beginning stages of the disease, a person's speech was coherent even if the subject matter was disorganized, in the end stages of the disease speech becomes progressively incoherent.

In addition to Alzheimer's disease, other forms of cognitive decline can impede a patient's ability to narrate his or her life coherently. Vascular events such as strokes can impair speech and neurological function, and degenerative diseases such as Parkinson's can similarly limit communication, though neurological abilities may remain stable or have the potential for improvement in such cases.[6] Additionally, a patient may present with dementia unspecified, a general diagnosis for cognitive impairment, typically used for elderly patients. Dementia is not a stand-alone disease, but an umbrella term for a constellation of symptoms such as memory loss and impaired capacity for daily function.[7] Alzheimer's disease is a form of dementia, the most prevalent type of dementia for those aged sixty-five to eighty-nine—the old, and ninety and above—the oldest-old.[8] While episodes of memory loss occur normally for aging patients, dementia is not understood to be a natural part of the aging process and is instead considered a form of damaged neurological function. A diminished ability to recall past events does not necessarily indicate dementia, such decline is typical and nonpathological.[9] In these cases of ordinary decline, prompts such as visuals or verbal reminders of either personal or historical events can rekindle a person's memory such that they can engage in the recollective process of life review. With patients who have dementia, the ability to understand verbal cues from another person deteriorates; therefore, direct questions posed to encourage reminiscence are less productive, though certain prompts may elicit a coherent, if mismatched, response, notably familiar music and ritualistic or mannered language such as an exchange of a greeting or farewell.[10]

Connections to Life Review

An Alzheimer's disease or dementia diagnosis does not entirely rule out the possibility of life review. For the majority of those affected, cognitive decline occurs gradually over time and, with an early diagnosis, a patient can intentionally engage in the process of life review with the knowledge that the ability to engage in lucid reminiscence will inevitability become impaired.[11] In a form of tailored care called "therapeutic environmental design" clinical attention centers on the parts of the brain, and the patient's abilities, that are functional rather than focusing on the capabilities that have been lost.[12] As Robert Butler noted in his seminal work on life review, the retrospective process is often prompted by a terminal diagnosis.[13] However, a diagnosis of dementia or Alzheimer's disease does not necessarily indicate that a person is imminently terminal (the six-month prognosis of death required by Medicare standards) and therefore eligible for hospice admission.[14] Thus, while a patient in the early stages of cognitive decline may have greater capacity to engage in the process of life review, they may be unaware of the process of formal retrospection or they may find the preparations for their eventual decline in cognitive and physical functionality to be more pressing than retrospective self-reflection.

The Loss of Socialization for Dementia Patients

In addition to memory loss and the loss of day-to-day functional abilities, those with dementia often experience a "social death."[15] One of the symptoms of the disease is a change in mood and presentation, and such dramatic changes can fragment relationships.[16] Furthermore, the patient may not recognize familiar and beloved friends and family members causing these individuals to minimize contact with the patient.[17] Because those with Alzheimer's disease and dementia are frequently unable to respond to another person's facial expressions or nuances in language, a growing estrangement can occur leading to isolation for the patient. Social distance can occur for various reasons: the caregiver may expect a give and take from the patient, a reciprocal dynamic that may not be possible due to the patient's disease.[18] Additionally, caregivers are often unpaid and provide care without adequate respite or social recognition or acknowledgement from the patient, all reasons why a caregiver may limit their role to providing the fundamentals of physical care to the patient.[19] Unfortunately, the patient can experience social neglect even if his or her medical and physical needs are being met.

Commendably, there are other forms of interaction for dementia patients that extend beyond a verbal framework. Art therapy, music therapy, dance, and other forms of creative self-expression are available to patients falling on a spectrum of cognitive and verbal ability.[20] Such modalities of self-expression do not rely on a patient's ability to offer a narrative arc of selfhood. Due to being more experiential in nature than results oriented, such activities may be more rewarding for patients whose cognitive capacities have declined, truly meeting them where they are and offering opportunities for stimulation, enrichment, and personal attention that extend beyond dialogical forms of personal interaction. Contemporary methods in narrative medicine seek to be patient-centered, creating an environment in which clinical caregivers tune in with patients and engage in rich dialogical exchange. However, the structure of the clinical encounter as framed by narrative medicine is one that excludes the growing population of patients with dementia. Additionally, the model of care in narrative medicine is dyadic in nature; however, a patient's experience extends beyond the one-on-one, clinician/patient model found in narrative medicine. The social experience of patients lacks salience in narrative medicine, due to a focus on a patient as a "character," a concern I address in the next section.

Individualism in Narrative Medicine

Some clinicians that align with the narrative medicine similarly address the individualism in narrative medicine and in medical ethics in general. Jack Coulehan notes:

> The first difficulty with the narrow focus on individuals in a doctor-patient relationship is that it distorts who an individual is in our society. Each of us is embedded in a complex matrix of relationships—family, friends, coworkers, churches, community. . . . Dyads are a convenient fiction in medical training,

but a fiction that distorts young physicians' understanding of the values inherent in their work.[21]

Because the words and gestures of dementia patients are often hard to interpret for those who may not be familiar with the patient, such as clinicians who have only episodic encounters with them, there is need to expand the dyadic nature of the clinical encounter as it exists in narrative medicine to a social model that includes those who know the patient. In so doing, the limits of narrative medicine can be addressed such that the model still has value for patients who may not be able to engage in lucid dialogue.

Social enactment is another form of communication for those with semantic dementia. Though they may be unable to articulate their ideas with language, some can convey meaning through acting out what they are trying to say.[22] Usually, this form of communication is most effective with those who are familiar with the patient, such as the patient's family or a medical staff member in a residential facility who frequently and informally interacts with the patient to the degree that the staff member can interpret the patient's verbal and nonverbal cues. Hyden and Orulv note that the storytelling engaged in by those with Alzheimer's disease can have a social and performative aspect. Caregivers familiar with the patient's stories can remind them of certain events and can serve as a responsive audience for the individual's account; they typically know the themes the patient values in the account and can support the development of the themes.[23] Dramatic arts are also useful for caregivers, usually nonclinical caregivers, in that the interaction enhances the bond a caregiver has with a patient, often a fraying bond due to caregiver burden.[24] Using drama has also proved efficacious as an educational tool for teaching clinicians how to understand and interact with dementia patients.[25]

MORAL IDENTITY AND LIFE REVIEW FOR VERBALLY AND COGNITIVELY COMPROMISED PATIENTS

How does one understand narrative selfhood after taking in the limits imposed by cognitive decline? In the following section, I address the dimensions of narrative selfhood that concern moral identity. Building on the last chapter, my specific research interest centers on moral inquiry as it manifests in life review for the elderly. However, in this chapter, taking into account those who have compromised ability to engage in verbal narration, my research expands to include other modalities of moral selfhood that include, but can move beyond, first-person written or spoken accounts of identity. As I argued in the last chapter, ethical reflection relies on a mode of narrativity that involves a reflexive turn, the ability to consider past behavior, and the ability to engage in self-reflection about such behavior through applying frameworks of moral reasoning, either implicitly or explicitly. This chapter includes other forms of identity expression that do not necessarily require the components needed for written or spoken life review.

Specifically, I identify categories of narrativity that include those who are able to recall events from their lives and can share these recollections with others as well as categories that can include patients with limited ability to communicate with others. To make distinctions between narrative capability for patients, specifically with regard to moral reflection, I use the terms agent narrativity, partial narrativity, and social narrativity, addressing how these categories of agency relate to moral identity in a narrative framework.

AGENT NARRATIVITY

Agent narrativity is the form of reflection such as that found in life review. Patients with agent narrativity are able to recollect events from their life and to reflect on these events, offering a moral evaluation of their circumstances or behavior, including missed opportunities or unfulfilled desires. They can do this independently, documenting their reflections in an autobiography or memoir, for instance. They can also do this in the form of structured life review with another person in which the person asks the patient questions and has the option of recording the response.[26] In such cases, it is the patient who is both the subject and the object of the analysis. They are the ones that generate the information, even if the remembrance is prompted or structured by another person, the other person functions in a secondary capacity as a catalyst for reminiscence. In agent narrativity, the patient can benefit from the presence of another person or a narrative structure that facilitates their memory, but it is not necessarily for the process of recollection and review. For verbally and cognitively challenged patients, however, their ability to engage in reflection requires assistance in the form of the guiding presence of another person or the cues provided by reminders such as memory books and music. I address the modalities of reminiscence when describing partial narrativity.

Moral Identity for Those with Agent Narrativity

Moral identity can be established in multiple ways. The topic draws on language that concerns selfhood: Who am I? Am I the person I aspired to be? How did I live? These questions become particularly salient for hospice patients facing the end of life. As established in chapter 3, patients often engage in this process of ethical analysis via life review, engaged in either formally or informally. Some take into account the entire narrative arc of their lives, while others reflect on their experience with a present-moment analysis. Though a person may not explicitly state that an ethical analysis is occurring, the presence of normative language—Was I a good father? Did I do what I wanted to do in life?—points to the activity of moral self-evaluation.

The interpretation of time comes into play in the process of life review; a patient engages in a self-assessment as the self functioned over time, with signposts in life marking significant events. Graduating high school, joining a religious body, starting a job, marrying one's spouse, all serve as points of remembrance for individuals reviewing their lives. These events may be signified through mementos around one's home or through photographs, and can prompt life review for patients able to independently engage in the process. In ways, these events can serve as "chapters" to a patient's life, upholding the narrative concept of identity as it relates to life review.

Time can function differently for patients depending on their residence. For patients who are at home, they may have more control over how time is structured day-to-day. Social markers of time such as birthdays and anniversaries can serve as external reminders of life events. For those living in a residential facility, however, time for ordinary events is not necessarily in the patient's control. The schedule of bathing, eating, and recreational, therapeutic, or medical activities may be designed to serve a multitude of patients with the goal of institutional efficiency rather than accommodating individual desires. Small, home-style residence models can offer an alternative to this institutional structure, allowing for more tailored care.

Additionally, the tenor of social relationships can change. Some Alzheimer's Disease patients experience the consequences of stigma when they disclose their diagnosis to friends, coworkers, and family members. Though their cognition may be declining, in the early stages of Alzheimer's Disease there remains an awareness of other's perception of one's status as cognitively impaired. Consequently, individuals with Alzheimer's Disease may be infantilized or avoided because of their diagnosis. John Turner notes that this is problematic because our identities are both internally and externally constructed; our sense of self cannot be fully separated from how we are perceived by others.[27]

With regard to self-analysis, however, previous research shows that patients are able to separate their individual sense of self from their socially recognized self, particularly when stigma is involved. For instance, when patients experience memory loss, even though this may cause distress in their caregivers or social group, the individual may interpret their experience as an aspect of typical aging, a nonpathological consequence of human development. This ability to separate one's self-appraisal from one's social-appraisal suggests that patients do retain a recognizable sense of identity, in the early stages of Alzheimer's Disease at least.

The process of life review shows moral analysis at work for verbal patients who have the requisite cognitive and verbal capacity to engage in the task. However, moral identity for verbally and cognitively challenged patients calls for closer attention. Though some scholars maintain that the self is fundamentally a narrative self, patients with Alzheimer's disease and patients with other forms of semantic dementia, though they may not have access to a linear store of memories, nevertheless demonstrate that they have a continuous sense of self.[28] Coherent use of first-person signifiers is present even for some in late-stage Alzheimer's Disease.[29] Additionally, there can also be periods of lucidity that indicate self-awareness.[30] Because patients claim that they have selfhood even though they cannot access all forms of selfhood (their married self or parental self, for instance) the question for consideration in such cases becomes, how then is moral analysis demonstrated for those with neurodegenerative status and a compromised ability to reflect on their lives?

PARTIAL NARRATIVITY

"Partial narrativity" is a term that recognizes those patients who may not able to engage in life review in a structured way but can still engage in reminiscence and reflection, both spontaneously and when prompted. In the following sections, I identify the multiple ways patients can engage in moral reflection even with verbal and cognitive limits. In the section following this one, I attend to forms of social narrativity that function even for patients who are mute, unconscious, or nonresponsive. Methods of social narrativity also apply to those who have died.

Moral analysis can occur for patients with early stage Alzheimer's disease; however, for advanced patients or for patients with mutism or those who cannot speak coherently, moral analysis can occur via proxy. This is also true for patients with full verbal and cognitive capacity; however, the observer's interpretation is then added to the patient's narrative, sometimes with the option of the patient correcting the content of either the observer's narrative or their own. With patients who are severely limited or who cannot speak, the narrative provided by the observer stands without the possibility of correction by the patient concerned. While someone who knows the patient may have access to more details of the person's life, a visitor may also be able to piece together elements of the person's moral identity through pictures, newspaper clippings, vocation, etc. This is all to say that the patient is not the exclusive source of moral analysis and that without the ability to self-interpret one's past behavior this behavior can nevertheless be interpreted socially.

Confabulation as an Example of Partial Narrativity

With Alzheimer's disease patients or patients with unspecified dementia, there are degrees of language ability, ranging from mild, moderate, to severe. Those on the advanced end of the spectrum with severe dementia may speak in gibberish or become mute and nonresponsive.[31] In mild to moderate forms of disease progression, patients do not completely lose access to communication; rather, their vocabulary becomes less nuanced, words are repeated, and their words may contain tendrils of truth or be true thematically, while not being historically true.[32] For instance, in her article "Making Sense of the Stories That People with Alzheimer's Tell: A Journey with My Mother," Jane Crisp identifies confabulation as a meaningful form of speech exhibited by Alzheimer's disease patients.[33] She draws on her conversations with her mother as representative of this type of speech. In confabulation, a patient blends past experiences or emotional states with their current experience. In her mother's case, her mother felt as though danger was near and she spoke of the loss of children. Her daughter initially thought that her mother was fabricating these stories, especially because of their fantastic nature. However, she came to realize that her mother lived by hot pools and there was a "danger" sign near them that she saw every day. She interprets her mother's language about the loss of children as pointing to the possibility that she had miscarriages that were not publically disclosed.

While Crisp's interpretations of her mother's account and other moves to interpret blended stories cannot necessarily be falsified or verified, such interpretations work to erode the notion that Alzheimer's disease patients are speaking nonsense and therefore do not call for being heard. Crisp listens to her mother's repeated concerns and responds with openness and compassion, recognizing that those with dementia are still aware of how they are perceived by others. There is call then to err on the side of listening to patients with dementia and attempting to interpret their language rather than dismissing their words as incoherent and disconnected from current reality. Crisp concludes in her research that family members often feel the impulse to correct patients and adjust the patient's claim to historical reality. She suggests that the impulse may originate from the observer's need to assert that they have uncompromised access to reality as it is.

Confabulation does not necessarily point to a process of ethical analysis, but, it does point to the existence of content-based language for compromised patients to such a degree that their speech is worth taking into account. Language that does point to ethical analysis is language of evaluation of one's earlier behavior. "I was a good x," "I was proud of x," "I should have done x," "if only," phrases such as these and their variants indicate moral self-analysis. Alzheimer's disease patients may not have full access to the entirety of their lives, though it is debatable whether persons without dementia have full access either. Regardless, the process of recollection and evaluation can still occur. This process can occur in structured fashion through life review or can happen spontaneously. Butler identifies both as modalities of life review.

Assisted Recall

Partial narrativity also manifests in the form of assisted recall. With assisted recall, patients are prompted to engage in reminiscence with visual or auditory aids. Depending on how advanced their deterioration is, the patient may have only minimal recollection of the events; however, the cues assist them in partial narration of their past behaviors. Because memory, specifically the details of past events, becomes impaired over time, with the initial diagnosis, a patient with agent narrativity can then work to make a document or visual collection that recounts the details of significant life events.[34] When the patient later experiences waning memory, the patient can be reminded of life events and either fill in the story or hear the story from others.

If no photos are available, caregivers can create generation scrapbooks based on the patients earlier context and time period in which they lived. With advanced dementia the patient may have no recollection of these events. Furthermore, the patient may show no discernible response to the person showing them the resource. A patient's flat affect can be difficult to encounter for visitors and caregivers who may be used to interpreting such a response as lack of interest. However, the social value of the interaction with the patient calls for engaging in the process even if the patient shows no recognition of the events in the book or does not demonstrate affirmative feedback about the process. Similar interactions could occur via video; however, because this is a more passive medium, the interaction may be less likely to occur. One of the benefits of video, however, is that a patient in early stages of dementia can record messages to their loved ones that can be used once the patient is no longer able to function at the same cognitive level. The benefit of using video in this way is that the person has a living record of the person in a multi-dimensional way—they can see them and their body language, can hear their voice. A moment in time is preserved as well.

In addition to scrapbooks, music has been successfully used to generate recollection in AD and other dementia patients. Music from a patient's earlier life can bring up memories of one's youth and young adulthood and evoke descriptions about that time period in a person's life. In addition to increasing cognitive activity, the process can also be therapeutic for patients in that the music serves as a form of companionship when other visitors are not present. Hospices often recognize the benefit of such therapies as scrapbooking and music and include them as part of the plan of care. Additional art therapies such as using color to describe emotion (with the assistance of small, colored stones among other physical aids) allow those who have an eroding vocabulary of words to describe their emotional state to nevertheless communicate information about their inner world. Such approaches are also useful in grief therapy to elicit responses in the bereaved that they may not be able to fully articulate or may not feel as though it is socially acceptable to feel. Music therapy in hospice can take the form of soothing music played at a patient's bedside to the use of music to facilitate relationality between patients and volunteers. Additionally, chaplains may be able to identify familiar hymns from a patient's faith tradition and play those for patients, offering comfort through deep familiarity.

Social media and other technological tools can also serve to facilitate recollection, evaluation, and social connection for patients.[35] Some AD patients begin blogging when they learn of their diagnosis so that they can record the experience and share it with others.[36] Real-time narration such as that which occurs via blogging can be an approach that includes moral reflection such as that found in life review. However, though it can be a more in-the-moment form of observation and appear to be stream of consciousness, if it is a public blog, a person may omit his or her moral self-analysis due to the potential of having a broad audience.[37] A person may instead offer an edited presentation of self rather than participating in a form of review that includes negative components of one's history and interpretations of moral identity.

In addition to social media, other forms of social support include groups in which AD patients meet with each other to talk about their experiences with the disease. Such groups can be more intimate because they are centered on those who have the disease (groups also exist for family members and caregivers of those who have the disease). Though my research on life review tends to have a retrospective focus, the social gatherings of those diagnosed with AD may be more oriented toward one's future self. Employing normative language, one can speak about the kind of person one wants to be and the kind of life one wants to have before and as they decline. This future orientation also represents a form of moral self-analysis in projected rather than review form.

Familiar Texts

The use of familiar texts can also facilitate partial review for patients. Favorite books from a person's childhood, familiar poems, sacred texts that they may have heard repeatedly, all can serve a therapeutic function, providing comfort even if the patient may have lost the ability to comprehend the meaning of the words. As with familiar hymns and common songs from the patient's earlier life, the rhythm of the language may be recognizable though the meaning is incomprehensible. Whereas the formal process of life review relies on the ability to access one's previous history, those engaging in the process can also draw on means of assistance such as those used in partial review. In so doing, the use of aids then does not become linked with a stigmatized disease and remains a neutral means of fostering reminiscence and possible reflection.

All of these forms of assisting recollection contribute a person's ability to demonstrate partial narrativity. The patient may not be able to bring forth a narrative account of his or her life when asked a direct question. However, prompts may facilitate dialogue and reflection on the part of the patient. When a patient has partial narrative ability, there can be moments of recognition from the patient that indicate a response of familiarity. However, even if no response occurs, the process nevertheless has therapeutic value for the patient because it involves social interaction, an activity that is repeatedly shown to decrease depression and agitation in patients.[38]

SOCIAL NARRATIVITY

Social narrativity relies exclusively on others speaking on behalf of the patient. In cases of social narrativity, the patient is physically or cognitively unable to speak and therefore is unable to express any form of retrospective moral analysis. However, a form of narrative identity still exists for such patient's. It can take the form of family members describing the patient as they knew them over time; it can also include the reports of coworkers who may have encountered another side of the patients' behavior. One form of social narrativity occurs by means of bereavement care for those surviving the patient's death. The hospice benefit offers one year of post-death bereavement care for family members and those close to the patient. In many cases, bereavement care begins before the patient dies. Doing so increases the likelihood that bereavement services will be used and creates a sense of continuity because those who cared for the patient continue to be available to share their experience with and memories of the person.

A concept of social narrativity allows for a concept of narrative identity to be viable even for patients who are unable to narrate. This mediates the concerns raised by figures such as Jerome Bruner who maintained that individuals who are unable to articulate a sense of self through narration do not have selfhood. Though Bruner did allow for a social understanding of narrativity, his primary interest was in a person being able to take into account the narration of another person, to be able to hear another as a separate individual. Without this ability, one's independent selfhood is compromised in his rubric. My understanding of social narrativity does not concern the ability to hear another's narrative as much as it concerns the observer's attempt to construct or recreate the narrative of another. It also includes the moral assessment of another's life according to one's terms as an observer. For instance, a son may say that he knew his mother identified as a good mother, but according to his expectations, his mother did not meet his social needs. Both appraisals are a form of social narrativity as it relates to moral identity.

The benefit of social narrativity is that it does not require functioning cognition on the part of the person being considered. A drawback is that the assessments cannot be verified by the person. They can, however, be verified by others who knew the person, other family members, other coworkers, other clinicians, and so forth. Moral analysis occurs through the interpretation of those who knew the individual. Ultimately, there is no one true moral assessment made by observers, or even by the individual person demonstrating agent narrativity for that matter.

One of the primary limits of narrative medicine is that the method of clinical care promoted in the model applies to a limited subset of the patient population. The patient has to be verbal and cognitively aware of self, others, and the environment around them, and they also need to have a retrospective sense of selfhood within time. Patients with semantic dementia are not taken into account in methods of narrative medicine because the model relies on a dialogical relationship between caregiver and patient. Ultimately, the patient has to be perceived as a rational agent for a narrative clinical encounter to operate. Rita Charon uses the language of mutuality and reciprocity to describe the equalization of roles within a clinical session framed by narrative medicine.[39] By focusing care on a portion of the patient population that has high-level cognitive abilities, other patients and their experiences can go unattended. Patients who cannot speak or think according to a level that corresponds with the clinician's expectations can be marginalized and rendered exempt from care.

CONTEXT OF CARE AND THE EFFECTS ON NARRATIVE PRACTICES

In this section, I address how the patient's context of care enhances or limits narrative methods in medicine, with special attention given to the process of life review for terminal adult patients. One's context of care, be it at home or in a hospital setting, crucially shapes the likelihood of this process occurring for patients. Specifically, I examine home-based care, hospital care, and residential care as areas that call for attention, as these are the contexts of care for most hospice patients. For hospital care and residential care, I identify different modalities of care within these contexts: acute care and standard care, such as the ICU and home-like or institutional facilities, respectively. Though the majority of patients claim to prefer receiving care and dying at home, hospice services and the location of death often occur in nonresidential contexts such as the intensive care unit.

In Robert Butler's research on life review, he claimed that older persons engage in a process of reflection about the course of their lives, particularly as they face life's end. He maintained that this is a universal feature of aging, one that is often prompted by a terminal diagnosis. I would add that an early diagnosis of Alzheimer's disease, Parkinson's disease, or other forms of neurodegenerative diseases can also move a person to reflect on and morally evaluate his or her life while they still have cognitive and verbal capabilities. As stated in chapter 2, I focus on hospice care because the model promotes direct conversation about the patient's impending death. This frankness about the patient's prognosis often leads to life review for a patient because they shift from a future concept of selfhood to a retrospective concept of selfhood. I suggest that the context of home-based care and home-like residential facilities offers the optimal living conditions for the manifestation of narrative moral identity through the process of life review when done informally. However, the formal process, because it is structured, limited, and timed, can be successfully undertaken regardless of context. While I include patients who have verbal and cognitive limitations, the patient population I address here is more general in scope.

Home Care

Hospice appeals to patients who prefer to remain at home in a familiar context with familiar caregivers. A benefit of remaining at home is that patients will receive personalized attention from a person who knows their history. In such cases, the likelihood of informal life review and individualized care may increase. However, patients can nevertheless go untended to by family members depending on their location in the home. For instance, if a patient is in a bedroom in the back of the house, he or she may only experience human contact when a specific need arises. One way to increase interaction with family life is to place the hospital bed in the living room of the home or another room where ordinary interactions occur. Doing so allows patients to be involved, even if through observation and physical presence, in the day-to-day household conversations. Having the patient's bed in the main room of the home may encourage family members to speak to the patient or to reminisce about the patient's life. Such encounters may prompt an informal process of life review for the patient.

For some patients, the possibility of unpaid, family caregivers there to provide continuous attention to their medical and nonmedical needs is not a realistic option. In such situations, paid caregivers can assist in a patient's activities of daily living and serve as a point person for the hospice care team. These more clinical relationships may not provide an ideal context for life review, as the caregiver is often paid by the hour to perform necessary care tasks such as bathing, feeding, and ambulating the patient. However, the nonfamilial relationship does not preclude a dialogical mode of relating for the patient and the caregiver; this relationship would exist on a case-by-case scenario depending on the desire and the personality of the patient and the personality of the caregiver.

Though prioritizing patient autonomy and preference with regard to many of the specifics of care, hospice is not a model that is fundamentally oriented to the individual patient. Admission requires the presence of a caregiver; only in exceptional cases will an independent patient be enrolled in hospice. The assumption is that as the patient declines, independent living will become untenable. The hospice care team, then, strives to prepare for the patient's future caregiving needs even if they are functioning sufficiently on their own when they are admitted.

If one is able to pay for their services, it is possible to have contingent caregivers provide assistance with the patient's daily needs. For some patients, however, a caregiver, either paid or unpaid, is a luxury that they do not have. Some patients may be homeless or not have a permanent home. Others may live alone for their safety, such as those enrolled in the Witness Protection Program, a program where a patient's former identity is "erased" and replaced with a new formal identity. In addition to having limited access to models of care such as hospice, the process of reminiscence and moral self-analysis that occurs in life review becomes complicated because the fractured nature of their lives.

Hospital Care

Though the majority of patients claim they would prefer to die at home either with unpaid or paid caregivers, deaths commonly occur in the hospital. This occurs for a variety of reasons; a patient may be receiving care at home, but when the person begins to actively die his or her caregivers will call an emergency number, rather than the on-call team in hospice. Additionally, a patient may experience a fall or an acute event such as a stroke that warrants a hospital admission and during this short-term stay the patient expires. There are some clear advantages to receiving end-of-life care in the hospital, a salient reason being that care is continuous and pain management options are immediately available. However, interactions in a hospital setting, particularly in an acute-care environment, are by necessity and design short and goal-oriented. Once the objective is achieved, for instance, administering a medication, the encounter ends without much opportunity for dialogue. An exception to this may be visits by nursing assistants there to take vital signs, an activity that allows for some level of verbal encounter that is not goal-based (conversations that occur while taking blood pressure, for instance). Physician Christine Puchalksi notes that it is often the janitor or the nursing assistant (roles that are seen as lower in the medical hierarchy) that the patient will speak to about his or her fears or desires, rather than the medical staff in the hospital.

In non-acute care contexts, such as the oncology unit in a hospital, opportunities to engage in repeated dialogical encounters are more likely to occur. One caveat is that hospice patients are unlikely to be in such environments because the model of care stipulates that patients receive no curative treatments. Some exceptions include treatments that sustain life, but do not prolong it, such as therapeutic radiation or dialysis treatments. Patients receiving daily care may be more likely to form relationships with clinical caregivers and hospital staff that they frequently see. Due to such day-to-day encounters, the possibility of a narrative process is more likely to occur. The patient can build a history with the person and they pick up where they left off in their next encounter. Additionally, the caregivers will then know the appropriate questions to ask to move into a more personal conversation with the patient. One of the limits of hospice is that these encounters are less likely to occur because of the model's limits on non-acute care. However, hospice visits for patients living at home or in long-term residential facilities allows for similar continuity of relationships with the hospice care team.

LONG-TERM RESIDENTIAL CARE AND OTHER CONTEXTS OF CARE

For patients who do not have family members, friends, or paid caregivers attending to their nonclinical medical and physical needs, the option of long-term assisted living facilities exists as an option for residential care. Additionally, patients can move to residential nursing units, though there can be time restrictions in such contexts because they are reimbursed by Medicare. With regard to narrative identity, a benefit of long-term residential care facilities is that they offer social opportunities for patients so inclined. A patient will have close neighbors living nearby and there is a higher chance for ongoing relationships to form. Furthermore, a patient's personal affects will be in the room (pictures, gifts, mementos, etc.) that can serve as prompts for conversation. Such contexts can provide an optimum environment for narrative identity to emerge. Unfortunately, long-term residential care facilities have few regulations in the United States and can function on a business model rather than one oriented to patient care. Many facilities also allow mentally and physically compromised patients to pay to live there when the patient needs a higher level of care than is provided in the residence. More research and oversight is called for when it comes to the management and goals of such facilities, especially with regard to patients who may require a higher level of care than is provided in long-term residential assisted living facilities.

Other Contexts of Care

Other contexts of care call for attention when it comes to analyzing moral identity for end-of-life patients. Not all patients have the benefit of caregivers or even of a permanent residence. Hospice does serve incarcerated patients; additionally, some prisons have fellow prisoners provide care and companionship for those who are terminal. However, for patients who are homeless or do not have a permanent home, care options are limited. Though patients may not be able to engage in the formal process of life review through the hospice model of care, bereavement services are available for those in community who knew the person. Through bereavement care a form of narrative construction of identity occurs. Utilization of such resources may be low, however, due to limited awareness about availability, financial constraints, transportation concerns, and other variables that limit access.

NARRATIVE IDENTITY IN THE CLINICAL ENCOUNTER TAKING CONTEXT INTO ACCOUNT

Narrative identity in the clinical encounter is more likely to flourish in the patient's home, a residential facility or in non-acute care wings in a hospital setting. The following conditions are conducive to the emergence of narrative moral identity through the process of life review: unstructured interactions, continuous relationships with caregivers, and relationships that exist over time. Fortunately, there are models of care structured to facilitate social interaction for patients who may not otherwise have it. For instance, in home-based environments, contexts intended to simulate a residential family-model, occasions such as conversations occurring while making a meal or doing the dishes can develop organically. The value of such conversations is that they are not limited to the medical structure expected in hospital care.

Hospice provides care for patients regardless of where they reside, though there is an expectation that the patient has a caregiver. Narrative identity is likely to manifest in hospice care because the model offers volunteer companionship for patients which will provide the unstructured interactions needed for narrative identity to manifest in the form of life review. Additionally, hospice provides spiritual care via professional chaplains who visit the patient in the patient's residence. While hospitals also provide chaplains, chaplains in the hospital context usually function in an on-call basis. Alternatively, pastoral care visits in the hospice model are often regularly scheduled, thereby allowing for both continuous relationships and for unstructured interactions. On an individual level, moral identity for hospice patients involves a process of evaluation centered on a fundamental ethics question: How did I live? Theologically, a patient may include what they perceive to be the perspective of the divine when they engage in this evaluative process. For instance, they may inquire as to whether they lived in a way that honored God, asking the question, "Did I live according to God's plans for me?" or they may feel deep guilt and regret at the recognition that God was aware of their ambiguous choices. Therefore, regular pastoral care visits can deepen a patient's moral inquiry, furthering the process of life review for patients. Hospice is a model that provides optimal conditions for narrative identity to emerge regardless of the patient's primary residence, be it at home or in a residential care facility.

CONCLUSION

Narrative methods in medicine (attending to a patient's story, parallel charting, life review, etc.) are valuable for some patients, but ultimately limited in scope, and often impractical given the growing population of those with dementia.[40] Not all patients are able to offer a self-narrative or understandable verbal response, due to a cognitive deficit such as Alzheimer's disease, aphasia, or lack of consciousness. Physically and cognitively some patients cannot think along the lines of a linear narrative and are unable to share their narrative with another. A patient with a cognitive deficit can also engage in behaviors that are interpreted by clinicians and caregivers, behaviors such as picking in the air or at themselves, nodding, rocking, staring, and other physical behaviors that may or may not have meaning. In a clinical context built on a dialogical model of patient-interaction, patients who are unable to meaningfully interact with others are needlessly forced into a position where they cannot adequately provide what the clinician seeks.

Expanding beyond narrative accounts that rely on verbal abilities, other forms of self-expression exist for patients that can supplement the dialogical model of narrative medicine, such as art-based therapies. Such therapies are also valuable because, as they do not rely on recollective storytelling. Rather, they allow a patient to be his or her current self, rather than focusing on a past sense of self, an aspect of identity that may be lost to the patient. Moving beyond a narrative-based patient encounter allows for greater patient involvement in comprehensive care in which a patient's experience is central. Additionally, methods of social narrativity in which those who know the patient and can speak about how the patient lived allows patients who cannot speak for themselves to benefit from attention given to their personal identity. This is particularly valuable for older patients, as many experience social isolation as they age.

Undoubtedly, narrative medicine can be mutually beneficial, both for caregivers who value the practice and for care receivers who value being heard. The model of care can create space for recognition, connection, and genuine relationality in a clinical context often described as impersonal. Training in the field can enhance a clinician's ability to attend very closely to what a patient is communicating, the premise being that a close reading of text correlates with detailed attention to patients, or, to use Ricoeur's language, methods in narrative medicine can create a context in which the "world of the text can meet the world of the reader." Many patients feel as though their personhood is overlooked by clinicians focused on physical care and efficiency.[41] The critique raised in this chapter is not intended to dispute the overall value of methods and training informed by the principles of narrative medicine, but to demonstrate the ways in which the approach is limited and can be supplemented by other models of engagement in and beyond clinical sessions.

Additionally, forms of person-centered care that do not rely on coherent verbal narration are available for patients who may not be able to engage in a dialogical clinical encounter. Forms of art therapy and social narrativity are accessible to a greater variety of patients, including those who are marginalized in narrative medicine, and patients do not have to perform in a context shaped by high-level dialogue. Such forms of care address many of the needs met narrative medicine, particularly the need for personal, individualized care. Due to the burgeoning demographic of those considered old (both "young-old" and "old-old"), there is reason to attend to the ways in which cognitive decline and compromised verbal ability intrude upon the ability to engage in narrative practice, including specified practices such as life review in hospice.

NOTES

1. Dementia is not a stand-alone diagnosis that makes one eligible for hospice care because a patient's decline can be gradual and is difficult to predict—a patient can have dementia for many years and not be terminally ill. However, many patients in hospice have a dual-diagnosis such as congestive heart failure and a form of dementia, and it is these patients that I take into account in this chapter.

2. "Alzheimer Deaths Increased during the Previous Decade," *JAMA* 309, no. 17 (May 1, 2013): 1767.

3. Alzheimer's Association, http://www.alz.org/alzheimers_disease_what_is_alzheimers.asp.

4. Life expectancy with Alzheimer's disease varies from three to ten years, with some living up to twenty-five years with the disease. Death usually occurs due to choking, falls, or infection, rather than cognitive decline. "2014 Alzheimer's Disease Facts and Figures," *Alzheimer's & Dementia* 10, no. 2 (2014): e59. However, current research shows that deaths due to dementia may be underreported: B. James, S. Leurgans, and L. Hebert et al., "Contribution of Alzheimer Disease to Mortality in the United States," *Neurology* 82 (2014): 1–6. Dying *with* dementia or *from* dementia is often a hard distinction to make. For more on the distinctions, see M. Ganguli and E. Rodriguez, "Reporting of Dementia on Death Certificates: A Community Study," *J Am Geriatr Soc* 47 (1999): 842–49.

5. Linda Örulv and Lars-Christer Hydén, "Confabulation: Sense-Making, Self-Making and World-Making in Dementia," *Discourse Studies* 8, no. 5 (2006): 647.

6. "2014 Alzheimer's Disease Facts and Figures." *Alzheimer's & Dementia* 10, no. 2 (3, 2014): e47.

7. Alzheimer's Association, http://www.alz.org/what-is-dementia.asp.

8. B. James, D. Bennett, P. Boyle, S. Leurgans, and J. Schneider, "Dementia from Alzheimer Disease and Mixed Pathologies in the Oldest Old," *JAMA* 307, no. 17 (2012): 1798.

9. The term for typical memory loss is mild cognitive impairment (MCI). While it can be an indicator of Alzheimer's disease, it does not always indicate a trajectory of further cognitive impairment. See the following text for more information, Glenn E. Smith and Mark W. Bondi, *Mild Cognitive Impairment and Dementia: Definitions, Diagnosis, and Treatment* (New York: Oxford University Press, 2013).

10. Mohamed El Haj, Virginie Postal, and Philippe Allain, "Music Enhances Autobiographical Memory in Mild Alzheimer's Disease," *Educational Gerontology* 38, no. 1 (2012): 30; Alison Wray, "Formulaic Language as a Barrier to Effective Communication with People with Alzheimer's Disease," *CMLR Canadian Modern Language Review/ La Revue Canadienne Des Langues Vivantes* 67, no. 4 (2011): 429. The latter article notes that the mannered or formulaic language used by patients does not always align with the structure of the conversation as understood by the caregiver and can lead to a caregiver choosing not to engage in further conversation with the patient.

11. Alzheimer's disease is categorized as either early-onset or late onset, depending on the age of the patient when diagnosed. The disease is then understood to be mild, moderate, or severe, with seven intermediate stages of decline, depending on the patient's symptoms. "Seven Stages of Alzheimer's," Alzheimer's Association, http://www.alz.org/alzheimers_disease_stages_of_alzheimers.asp. The framework was developed by physician Barry Reisberg. The following article is by Reisberg et al, "Stage-Specific Behavioral, Cognitive, and In Vivo Changes in Community Residing Subjects with Age-Associated Memory Impairment and Primary Degenerative Dementia of the Alzheimer Type," *DDR Drug Development Research* 15, no. 2–3 (1988): 101.

12. M. Friedrich, "Therapeutic Environmental Design Aims to Help Patients with Alzheimer Disease," *JAMA* 301, no. 23 (June 17, 2009): 2430.

13. Robert Butler, "The Life Review: An Interpretation of Reminiscence in the Aged," *Psychiatry* 26 (1963): 65.

14. K. Yaffe, "Treatment of Alzheimer Disease and Prognosis of Dementia: Time to Translate Research to Results," *JAMA* 304, no. 17 (2010): 1952–53. The authors note that prognostic tools that would allow patients with dementia to be admitted to hospice are still in development. At this point, the rate of decline is too variable to accurately determine a diagnostic window that would make patients with dementia hospice eligible. For more information on the development of a prognostic tool, see the following: S. Mitchell, S. Miller, and J. Teno et al., "Prediction of 6-Month Survival of Nursing Home Residents with Advanced Dementia Using ADEPT vs Hospice Eligibility Guidelines," *JAMA* 304, no. 17 (2010): 1929–35.

15. Helen Sweeting and Mary Gilhooly, "Dementia and the Phenomenon of Social Death," *SHIL Sociology of Health & Illness* 19, no. 1 (1997): 93.

16. "2013 Alzhiemer's Disease Facts and Figures, Symptoms of Alzhiemer's Disease," Alzhiemer's Association.

17. Thomas Kitwood drew attention to the social aspects of dementia, emphasizing that they can often be just as, if not more, debilitating that the neurological and physical aspects of the condition. Tom Kitwood, "The Dialectics of Dementia: With Particular Reference to Alzheimer's Disease," *Ageing & Society* 10, no. 2 (1990): 177; T. M. Kitwood, *Coping with Dementia: The Person Comes First* (Leicester: British Psychological Society, 1996); Jan Dewing, "Personhood and Dementia: Revisiting Tom Kitwood's Ideas," *OPN International Journal of Older People Nursing* 3, no. 1 (2008): 3.

18. Satisfaction can come from providing care to patients—the experience, while challenging, is not wholly negative. Adult children serving as informal caregivers for parents experience less satisfaction from providing care than do spouses. See the research of M. Lawton et al., for research on the subject: "A Two-factor Model of Caregiving Appraisal and Psychological Well-Being," *Journals of Gerontology* 46, no. 4 (1991): 181–89.

19. H. Kim, M. Chang, K. Rose, S. Kim, "Predictors of Caregiver Burden in Caregivers of Individuals with Dementia," *Journal of Advanced Nursing* 68, no. 4 (2012): 846.

20. B. Chancellor, A. Duncan, A. Chatterjee, "Art Therapy for Alzheimer's Disease and Other Dementias," *Journal of Alzheimer's Disease : JAD* 39, no. 1 (2014): 1; Heather Hill, "Journey without a Map: Dance Therapy with Dementia Patients," *How the Arts make a Difference in Therapy* (1993), 89; D. Duignan, L. Hedley, R. Milverton, "Exploring Dance as a Therapy for Symptoms and Social Interaction in a Dementia Care Unit," *Nursing Times* 105, no. 30 (2009): 4.

21. Jack Coulehan, et al., "The Best Lack All Conviction: Biomedical Ethics, Professionalism, and Social Responsibility," *Cambridge Quarterly of Healthcare Ethics* 12, no. 1 (2003): 24.

22. Jacqueline Kindell, Karen Sage, John Keady, and Ray Wilkinson, "Adapting to Conversation with Semantic Dementia: Using Enactment as a Compensatory Strategy in Everyday Social Interaction," *JLCD International Journal of Language & Communication Disorders* 48, no. 5 (2013): 497.

23. L. Hyden and L. Orulv, "Narrative and Identity in Alzheimer's Disease: A Case Study," *Journal of Aging Studies* 23, no. 4 (2009): 209.

24. Margret Lepp, Karin Ringsberg, Ann-Kristin Holm, and Gunilla Sellersjö, "Dementia – Involving Patients and Their Caregivers in a Drama Programme: The Caregivers' Experiences," *JOCN Journal of Clinical Nursing* 12, no. 6 (2003): 873.

25. Pia Kontos and Gary Naglie, "Expressions of Personhood in Alzheimer's Disease: An Evaluation of Research-Based Theatre as a Pedagogical Tool," *Qualitative Health Research* 17, no. 6 (2007): 799.

26. Barbara K. Haight and Barrett S. Haight, *The Handbook of Structured Life Review* (Baltimore: Health Professions Press, 2007).

27. John C. Turner, *Rediscovering the Social Group: Self-Categorization Theory* (Oxford, UK; New York, NY: B. Blackwell, 1987).

28. L. Tippett and D. Addis, "Memory of Myself: Autobiographical Memory and Identity in Alzheimer's Disease," *Memory (Hove, England)* 12, no. 1 (2004): 57.

29. R. Tappen, C. Williams, S. Fishman, and T. Touhy, "Persistence of Self in Advanced Alzheimer's Disease," *Image: Journal of Nursing Scholarship* 31 (1999): 121–25.

30. H. Normann, K. Asplund, and A. Norberg, "Confirmation and Lucidity during Conversations with a Woman with Severe Dementia," *Journal of Advanced Nursing* 39 (2002): 370–76.

31. Wray, *Formulaic Language as a Barrier to Effective Communication with People with Alzheimer's Disease*, 429–58.

32. Ibid.

33. Jane Crisp, "Making Sense of the Stories That People with Alzheimer's Tell: A Journey with My Mother," *Nursing Inquiry* 2, no. 3 (1995): 133.

34. Baddeley et al. use the language of "clouding" to describe the loss of detail that occurs for those with dementia: "Dementia and Working Memory," *Quarterly Journal of Experimental Psychology* 38A (1986): 603–18.

35. J. Rodriquez, "Narrating Dementia: Self and Community in an Online Forum," *Qualitative Health Research* 23, no. 9 (2013): 1215.

36. For instance, "Silverfox" blogs about his experience with Lewy body dementia due to Parkinson's disease: http://parkblog-silverfox.blogspot.com/. The blog creates

a record of narrative self-expression, shows how he copes with his changing cognitive state, and serves as a vehicle for social interaction as he can see how many people have viewed his site and can interact with readers via comments and email.

37. A benefit of the publicness of online social media is that it can connect individuals to each other who may otherwise be isolated as their disease progresses. Online support groups are also valuable for caregivers of those with dementia who may be unable to physically leave the patient alone to attend in-person support groups. Alzheimer's Association, "Caregivers Support Groups," http://www.alz.org/care/alzheimers-dementia-support-groups.asp.

38. Additional forms of supplemental therapies include massage and pet therapy. While valuable for sensory stimulation and social interaction, these were not addressed directly as they do not designed to create opportunities for narrative self-reflection. L. West and J. Polubinski, "Implementation of a Massage Therapy Program in the Home Hospice Setting," *Journal of Pain and Symptom Management* 30, no. 1 (2005): 104; M. Maleske, "Hospice Care. Pet Therapy," *Hospitals & Health Networks/AHA* 78, no. 11 (2004).

39. Rita Charon, "Narrative Reciprocity," *Hastings Center Report* 44, no. 1 (2014): S21.

40. Rita Charon, "Narrative Medicine: Form, Function, and Ethics," *Annals of Internal Medicine* 134, no. 1 (2001): 83–87.

41. D. E. Epner and W. F. Baile, "Patient-Centered Care: The Key to Cultural Competence," *Annals of Oncology* 23, no. suppl 3 (April 1, 2012): 33.

Chapter 5

Expanding beyond Narrative

Hospitality, Accompaniment, and Companioning as Models of Presence with Patients

Practices in narrative medicine, such as life review and the conversations prompted by spiritual assessments, can enrich the clinical relationship between patients and their clinical caregivers. Yet many patients are unable to engage in substantial conversation with their clinicians due to cognitive impairments. Such patients are at risk of experiencing social isolation because they do not have the capacity to interact in reciprocal, verbally coherent dialogue. Expanding beyond narrative practices, there is a need for ways of engaging with patients who are confused or unable to speak. In this chapter, I identify ways of being with patients who do not require the higher-level verbal and cognitive abilities necessary for dialogical interaction in the clinical encounter. These practices include both religious approaches to care for others and nonreligious practices of care.

Narrative medicine serves as a meaningful form of engagement for clinicians and patients who have the verbal capacity to participate in dialogue. Here I discuss the ways clinicians can be present with patients who may not be able to respond verbally in the clinical encounter. I suggest a retrieval of religious modes of being and practices for both hospice patients and caregivers, looking to how the theological concept of hospitality can accommodate those in pain and those experiencing discomfort, uncertainty, or grief. I examine a selection of practices that I suggest are portrayals of hospitality. The selection of practices is not meant to be comprehensive, but to show how multiple approaches to pain can be interpreted as demonstrating hospitality. For caregivers, the religious practice of bearing witness, as articulated here by Dorothee Soelle, serves as an example of how one can be present for patients regardless of their cognitive or verbal abilities.

The practice of accompaniment described by Paul Ricoeur in *Living Up to Death* reflects a similar approach to being with patients, particularly those at the end of life. Another option, "companioning the dying" described by grief counselor Greg Yoder, offers a way of being with patients, similar to Ricoeur's, that can be practiced by those who identify as spiritual or religious as well as those who are nonreligious. Though the concept has religious roots, hospitality does not have to be interpreted or practiced from a theological point of view.[1]

PAUL RICOEUR'S MEDITATION ON THE END OF LIFE

In Ricoeur's text *Living Up to Death*, Paul Ricoeur presents a meditation on death and describes a mode of being with those who are dying that does not rely on narrative capacities or dialogical interaction. Ricoeur began writing *Living Up to Death* in 1996 as his partner of sixty-three years, Simone Ricoeur, was physically declining.[2] He set aside his work on the text to attend to her and, after her death, did not return to the text for another eight years. His own health began to decline and, though he continued to work on the text and edit *Course of Recognition*, his growing weakness and fatigue caused him to focus less on his writing work. His experience at the end of life shows a transition from narrative-based activity, writing and conversation, to a time of refection and encounter with the arts. Catherine Goldenstein writes, "[H]e tried as long as possible to 'be there, alive' through reading, following the news, receiving a few friends as visitors, looking forward to conversation, and, once speaking itself became difficult, by listening to music."[3] *Living Up to Death* was published posthumously and contains fragments of text that he wrote during the last few months of his life as well as his reflections on how to be present with others as they are dying, which he wrote during his wife's decline.

In the section on how to be present with others, Ricoeur identifies a mode of being with the dying that is not focused on the person as a being-toward-death, in the vein of Heidegger, but rather as a person that lives up to death. From his conversation with palliative care physicians, he makes two conclusions: "First, this: so long as they remain lucid, ill, dying people do not see themselves as dying, as soon to be dead, but as still living," and, "Next, again this: what occupies one's still preserved thoughts is not concern for what there is after death, but rather the mobilization of the deepest resources of life to still affirm itself."[4] Ricoeur suggests that one be present with a dying person with an approach based on beholding the person as living rather than as dying. Approaching a person this way is fundamental to the practice of what he calls accompanying, a mode of being with patients, centered in compassion, that honors their experience living up to death.

Ricoeur recognizes that the end of life can be a profoundly spiritual time, one that is not limited to the strictures of organized religion, but one that is focused on what Ricoeur calls the essential. He says, "[W]hat the physician in the palliative care unit bears witness to is the grace granted some dying people that assures what I have called the mobilization of the deepest resources of life in the coming to light of the Essential, fracturing the limitations of the conventionally religious."[5] Ricoeur maintains that accompanying a person as they face death involves honoring the spiritual dimension of their experience, an experience that cannot be known from the outside. Ricoeur recommends a mode of being with patients modeled on the giving-receiving involved in friendship and a gaze of compassion and understanding that the person is still living. He says:

> I come back to the nonmedical quality of the gaze and above all to the gesture of accompanying. It indicates the fusion, in the hermeneutics of the medicine of palliative care, between understanding and friendship. The understanding is directed toward the life coming to an end and its recourse to the essential. The friendship helps not just the person dying but this understanding itself.[6]

In *Living Up to Death*, Ricoeur considers the idea of death and the event of death, but he does not write in the abstract about the experience of caring for others at the end of life. Instead, he focuses on what it means to be with another person as they transition. Ricoeur's words speak about the value of being present with those who are facing death, rather than leaving them to decline and die alone.

In her research and clinical work in hospice care, Cicely Saunders also spoke about the value of physical presence with the dying. As a narrative source for her perspective on the value of presence for the dying, she looks to the experience of Jesus of Nazareth the night before his death, who asks that his friends remain awake with him, to watch with him:

> I am sure the most important foundation stone we could have comes from the summing up of all the needs of the dying which was made for us in the Garden of Gethsemane in the simple words "Watch with me." I think the one word "watch" says many things on many different levels, all of importance to us. In the first place it demands that all the work at St. Christopher's should stem from respect for the patient and very close attention to his distress. It means really

looking at him, learning what this kind of pain is like, what these symptoms are like, and from this knowledge finding out how best to relieve them.[7]

Both Ricoeur and Saunders speak about how one is attuned with the dying person, attending to the person in a deep, personal way rather than with clinical detachment or an exclusive focus on physical pain management. Cicely Saunders recognized the human experience of health care, seeing that pain is not merely physical, it has personal, social, and spiritual dimensions. One of her first patients, David Tasma, a forty-year-old man with terminal cancer, suffered not only because of his physical illness, but also because of the non-medical elements of his experience: his foreshortened future, a sense of a life unlived, and the profound loneliness that can accompany those who go unvisited as they face death. Tasma, a Jewish immigrant from Poland, resided in England in his final years, separated from his family, friends, and religious community. He knew few people in England. Saunders visited him and formed a deep sense of connection with him as a person, a relationship that transcended that of clinician-patient, and a relationship that inspired her to found the first formal hospice center, St. Christopher's, in London. Her care for him was healing, but it was not primarily medical. Saunders's care for Tasma was relational, dialogical, and spiritual. Their time together was spent in conversation about his state of being, reflecting a narrative-based, dialogical encounter.

In addition to valuing the spiritual and psychosocial dimensions of health care, Saunders recognized that pain calls for more than just pharmacological treatment. The distress Tasma experienced was social and existential, and it is this experience of pain, what Saunders calls "total pain," that health care chaplains are trained to address. A health crisis can elicit paralyzing feelings of fear and threaten a person's sense of security and identity. A person experiencing a health crisis, and the emotional and social pain that follows in its wake, needs someone to listen to as they navigate their new landscape of being. Having a chaplain available for emotional and existential support is invaluable in such circumstances. Essentially, a person needs someone to be there with them in their suffering. In a section called "Being There" in her 1965 book *Watch with Me*, Saunders says the following:

> "Watch with me" means, still more than all our learning of skills, our attempts to understand mental suffering and loneliness and to pass on what we have learnt. It means also a great deal that cannot be understood. Those words did not mean "understand what is happening" when they were first spoken. Still less did they mean "explain" or "take away." However much we can ease distress, however much we can help the patients to find a new meaning in what is happening, there will always be the place where we will have to stop and know that we are really

helpless. It would be very wrong indeed if, at that point, we tried to forget that this was so and to pass by. It would be wrong if we tried to cover it up, to deny it and to delude ourselves that we were always successful. Even when we feel that we can do absolutely nothing, we will still have to be prepared to stay. (1965, 4)

Both Saunders and Ricoeur describe modes of being with patients that do not require narrative capacities on the part of the patient. Narrative medicine focuses on the dialogical features of person-centered clinical care and the practices involved in narrative medicine develop the ability to pay close attention to a patient's narrative experience. Clinicians and health care chaplains can draw on methods in narrative medicine to engage with patients on an intimate, personal level. However, there are patients who are unable to participate in meaningful, reciprocal dialogue due to physical or cognitive limits. With such patients, attentive presence is still beneficial, particularly for those who are socially isolated, but the encounter cannot rely only on verbal ability. There is a need for other forms of presence with patients that expand beyond narrative approaches to clinical care.

Clinicians working with patients at the end of life may find themselves uncomfortable meeting with patients who are nonverbal or cognitively challenged. By the time patients are enrolled in hospice care, many are unable to engage in meaningful dialogue with their clinicians or to participate in narrative practices such as life review. Hospice practitioners visit patients who are nonresponsive, and may have the impression that there is little need to spend time with patients who are nonverbal and appear to be unaware. As we see from the work of Saunders and Ricoeur, a caregiver does not have to be demonstrating high-level clinical skills for patients at the end of life for their time to be worthwhile. Merely being with patients in a spirit of compassion and attentive regard can meet the needs of patients for presence at the end of life.

HOW RELIGION CAN ADDRESS THE LIMITS OF NARRATIVE METHODS IN MEDICINE WITH NONVERBAL PATIENTS

Life review and spiritual assessments can serve as useful prompts for conversations about religion that otherwise may not occur in the clinical encounter. However, such tools suffer from the same limits of narrative medicine addressed in chapter 4. While maintaining the value of life review and spiritual assessments for patients who are verbal and cognitively able to engage in such activities, I recognize that not all are able to offer a coherent narrative of selfhood or spiritual or religious identity due to limitations often related to their decline. For instance, they require a degree of self-reflection that may not be available to patients in pain. Narrative methods, by design, rely on a high level of awareness and ability for patients, a level that may not be possible for patients at the end of life. Additionally, spiritual assessments assume that the patient is able to speak about his or her history, community, and beliefs.

I suggested previously that life review as it manifests in hospice care demonstrates a process of moral self-analysis. A person, when faced with the end of his or her life and when equipped with the cognitive ability, makes a retrospective turn and evaluates how he or she lived. One of the dimensions or moral self-evaluation concerns religion and spirituality. A patient may consider whether or not he or she lived in a way that honored God; additionally, a patient may feel abandoned or judged by God. Limiting life review to a mere recounting of biographical events impoverishes a process that is intended to be a mode of reflection about what mattered most for patients. For many, there are religious or spiritual aspects of their identity that call for attention, such aspects of selfhood can go unrecognized by secular models of care. Frequently talk about the role of religion in medicine approaches religious and spiritual care as ad hoc, a supplemental form of add-on care that enhances a patient's experience in and beyond the clinical encounter. A person's religious identity is rarely just an accent to who they are, however. Instead, religiosity can deeply inform how a person views his or her identity and experience of illness and suffering. It also offers a frame for interpreting the totality of a person's life, body, mind, and spirit. In the next section, I examine hospitality as a theological frame for a concept of presence with patients that includes, but expands beyond, narrative-based models of patient care.[8]

HOSPITALITY AS A PRACTICE FOR HOSPICE PATIENTS AND CAREGIVERS

The word hospital and the word hospice share the same etymological source: the root word *hoste*, a word that means both guest and host.[9] From this source, the word "hospitality" is derived, a word that connotes positive reception of guests. All three of these terms, hospital, hospice, and hospitality concern relationships with the stranger, in some cases the unbidden, unwelcome stranger. The concept of hospitality connects with medical care by offering an alternative medical epistemology, particularly for dying patients. In this section, I attend to the ways a theological concept of hospitality can function for both hospice patients and caregivers.

In addition to the recognition of spiritual pain fundamental to the hospice model of care, there is also a recognition of the grotesque body, or the body as stranger. In hospice, honesty about what to expect in the dying process shapes conversations in the clinical encounter. Without softening content, patients and caregivers are informed about potential social and physical changes the patient may experience. Contrary to the image of the deathbed gathering—the sentimentalized notion of the "good death"—socially, a patient may turn inward and become uninterested in life events like anniversaries, birthdays, and graduations. As the person moves closer to death there are also marked physical changes; skin may become cold and feel moist, toes and lips may turn blue or purple, breathing may appear labored and sound like gasping or a rattle. A beloved person can become unfamiliar or may not recognize friends and family members; they may become like strangers to each other.

Turning to a theological analysis, it is hospice's hospitality to the body as stranger that demonstrates the model's contribution to medical epistemology. In the New Testament, the Greek word *philoxenia* is used in reference to hospitality in the early Christian tradition. The roots of this word are *philieo*, a love of those who are known to us and for whom we have friendly affection, and *xenos*, the word for stranger.[10] Hospitality, thus, is not about providing sustenance for beloved family and friends; rather it is about providing the type of care that we would show to family or close friends to then meet the needs of those who are foreign to us. To make the distinction it may help to understand hospitality as serving as host to the alien rather than as offering welcome to the wanted and expected guest.[11] Because the language of hospitality connotes delight at the visitor's presence, using the term "hosting" instead allows for the recognition that the experience of encountering the stranger is not necessarily a positive one in which one greets the stranger with kindness and offers a gift of welcome. With regard to the role of the caregiver, a theological understanding of hospitality as hosting means that the focus is on the guest and not on the host as the gracious bestower of gift. The concept of hosting suggests creating space for another with no expectation of reciprocation or recognition.

In his text *Anatheism*, Richard Kearney claims that one can respond to the call of the stranger in two ways, with hospitality or with hostility.[12] However, because the stranger possibly bears the presence of the divine, he urges one to risk responding to the stranger's call with hospitality rather than hostility, opening oneself up to encountering the sacred in the form of the stranger. Kearney's work can deepen an understanding of how to live with pain, particularly pain that extends over time and cannot be managed pharmacologically. Building on his work, pain can be interpreted as the uninvited, even unwelcome, stranger that demands a response. The "stranger" is not necessarily separate from us; rather, when one experiences bodily pain one can perceive one's own body as a site of alienation, even invasion. Rather than responding with hostility, which I interpret as aggressive medical care, one can respond with hospitality, serving as a host to an unwelcome guest. Hosting is a particularly valuable concept with regard to how terminal patients respond to pain, particularly pain that cannot be fully managed medically, such as the "total pain" Saunders describes. Hosting presents a way for patients to maintain agency during a time when much is out of their control and the possibility of the complete erasure of pain is minimal or, for some, undesired. The concept of hosting pain does not involve militaristic approaches to clinical care or sacrificially enduring pain; instead, hosting pain can be interpreted as allowing a strange presence to exist within you without having to strenuously fight this presence or having to warmly greet it.

Before speaking about what it means to host pain as the stranger, let me briefly outline what hostility looks like in the medical model of care. In the biomedical model of care in the United States, war-based language is often used to frame a plan of care or conversation about symptom management. There is a "battle to be won," a patient chooses to "fight," a tumor will be "destroyed," disease is the "enemy," and ultimately death is a "foe" to be fought as well.[13] The Dylan Thomas line "Rage against the dying of the light" is used as a rallying cry. This approach to pain management—hostility—values agency, power, and resistance. While there is merit in this approach, it can be employed needlessly for patients for whom it is more costly, physically, emotionally, and socially, than it is beneficial. For instance, if a patient has to leave one's family to receive specialized medical care in another city, and this patient has a terminal prognosis and limited energy, the personal cost of treatment in terms of separation from a support network and the energy it takes to participate in medical treatment can dramatically outweigh the benefits. What is the value of fighting the "battle" against disease when one is alone, exhausted, and exiled from home?

Denial of illness is another form of hostility. Hostility is not limited to aggressive forms of treatment; it can also include neglect of self and others. Rather than neglect being an absence of agency, it is an intentional choice not to act in the interest of wellness. In medicine, this would manifest in the form of not following through with the clinical plan of care, or not heeding the call of the body to receive medical attention. There is one asterisk here that calls for attention and that is that social minorities, including, but not limited to those who are marginalized due to size, gender, class, race, or ability, often are shaped to believe that their bodies are not valuable and therefore do not warrant care. Finally, a third form of hostility toward pain is to hide the broken body in a cocoon of technology. When one is hidden in what is thought to be the necessary and protective barrier of medical equipment, there is distance created between the body as-it-is and the body as shielded from the reality of pain, disease, and death. Concealing the compromised body can be perceived as a form of hostility toward the body.

The option of hospitality, in which one sees oneself as a host to the stranger, does not require an aggressive posture, or a charitable one. By hosting the pain residing within you, there is no expectation that one has to cheerfully greet this presence or that one has to fight it. Instead, one recognizes its presence and makes accommodations for it. By making accommodations, one engages in all forms of pain management available, including pharmacologic treatments. Hosting pain does not mean passively accepting its presence; it instead means recognizing the limits of one's ability to remove it. With chronic pain related to terminal disease, daily treatment for pain may limit one's ability to be aware to such a degree that the burdens outweigh the benefits of medical treatment. Furthermore, not all pain can be treated pharmacologically. Though hospice and palliative care physician Ira Byock maintains that all physical pain can be treated, not all pain is located in the body; spiritual and emotional pain can remain even when one's physical pain is managed.[14] Additionally, a person may not want to turn to pharmacologic treatments due to medical side effects such as fatigue or nausea or because they are unable to access the financial or medical resources to fully manage their pain. Because not all forms of pain can be or are ameliorated medically, in addition to responding to the stranger with hostility or hospitality, hosting offers another type of response, one that stands as a mediating point between welcome and rejection.

One may not be able to make the pain leave; however, one can maintain agency through how the presence of pain is interpreted. When one is unable to exercise power over the presence of pain in the body, one can still, assuming cognitive ability remains, have agency in how one responds to pain. Though pain can involve a disruption of self that causes one to feel dispossessed, through communicating one's pain to others, one can hold to a sense of self through the witness of another who recognizes the pain one is hosting. Dorothee Soelle in her text *Suffering* describes the agency involved in identifying, naming, and articulating to another the conditions of one's suffering.[15] According to Soelle, suffering is compounded when experienced alone and suffering is reduced when its reality is communicated to and recognized by another.

DOROTHEE SOELLE ON SUFFERING, LANGUAGE, AND BEARING WITNESS

In Soelle's text, she offers a resource for how to interpret and respond to physical, mental, social, and spiritual pain from a Christian standpoint, though her claims are not limited to this tradition. Rather than looking at suffering in a monochromatic way, she looks at different types of suffering with particular attention given to suffering that is caused by human agents. She presents two primary questions: "What are the causes of my suffering?" and "What meaning can be found in my suffering?" She examines Christian responses to these questions, particularly responses that she sees as limited or even dangerous. For instance, the idea that God intentionally sacrificed God's child out of love is a concept of God that has consequences for human behavior, one that can increase suffering rather than freeing Christians from it.[16] Even the idea of a suffering God can be problematic, particularly if it leads one to passive resignation to suffering, both suffering in one's own life and in the lives of others.[17] Any spiritualization of suffering that limits human agency is one she will unapologetically critique. For Soelle, suffering that is caused by political or economic social conditions does not call for passive acceptance, denial, or resting in "meaning." Rather, it calls for intentional effort oriented toward social transformation in a way that honors God.

In terms of a model for how to respond to suffering, the theologically informed process of articulation Soelle describes can lead one from passivity to transformative agency in response to suffering. The first response is being rendered mute by suffering and being utterly paralyzed in the face of one's experience. The second response is moving to a place of lament. One way of engaging in lament is through using psalmic language. Psalms can also serve as a source for participating in communal responses to suffering, supplementing one's individual response to both the experience of pain and the relationship one has with sacred texts. Finally, Soelle's third step is to engage in acts of social transformation in which one works to eliminate the conditions that cause suffering. While the third movement in Soelle's process is less germane to hospice patients, it nonetheless can be understood as a way to respond to pain management, with the focus on reducing or eliminating pain through medical, psychosocial, and spiritual modes of care.

Soelle's theological orientation emerges in her mystical understanding of suffering and selfhood—that there is a type of union with God that occurs in which one's self becomes incorporated in the mystery of God's self. Though as a Christian realist, Soelle could be seen as being suspicious of how the language of "mystery" is used and how this language functions as another form of passivity, she does use language of the void in a way that is similar to the poetic language of mystery. Drawing on the work of Simone Weil, Soelle notes that suffering can be a time when one can touch the limits of the void of human experience.[18] It is through the act of loving even in the void that one can have agency within suffering. In hospice, there is awareness that death is a limit of life, similar to the limit of the void, and it is through recognition of and preparation for this limit that patients and family members can have agency and can experience death in its fullness, not necessarily as a positive event, but as a natural one in the course of human life.

In addition to offering the model of naming and articulating one's pain through lament, Soelle offers another mode of response: one can bear witness to pain. Bearing witness is something one can do particularly in response to the suffering of another. However, one can bear witness to the pain that dwells within oneself as well, a theological variation of hosting. One can recognize the pain or grief that inhabits one's being, without having to work to obliterate this presence through aggressively curative medical care such as that provided in the biomedical model or having to amiably endure it in a posture of welcome or benign passivity. Both the model of bearing witness and Soelle's three-phase response to pain demonstrate Kearney's vision of how one can be host to the "unwelcome guest" of pain, particularly the physical, emotional, and spiritual pain experienced by terminal patients in hospice.

A THEOLOGY OF HOSPITALITY FOR HOSPICE CAREGIVERS

In discourse about medicine and religion, attention often centers on the religious or spiritual identity of the patient as the recipient of care. Respect for patient's rights and a mission of patient-centered humanistic care motivate a clinician's attention to take into account the patient's identity in its fullness; such an approach includes recognition of dimensions of patient identity that incorporate spiritual and the religious aspects of selfhood that prove significant for a sizable majority of patients. In this section, I reframe the conversation. Rather than turning toward the patient's religious or spiritual identity as is so often done in research on religion and medicine, I turn toward the religious and spiritual identity of the caregiver. Rather than addressing the spiritual or religious identity of the caregiver, previous research has centered on the spiritual and religious role of the caregiver; however, that research continues to be patient-oriented in that it focuses on how to best provide care for patients, usually through an initial spiritual assessment prompted by the clinician. Instead of a role orientation, in which a clinician attunes to the needs of the patient, I consider the ways in which a clinician's spiritual or religious identity can provide a way of interpreting and engaging in the practice of care. I propose that a theology of hospitality can be a resource for how a caregiver approaches care for a person at the end of life. In the following section, I speak about how theology offers both a frame for understanding how a caregiver approaches patient care and a modality of care for those who are dying.

The theological concept of hospitality connects with the early history of the hospice movement in the West. Hospices provided a place of respite for soldiers, the indigent, or those on pilgrimage, the work perceived as a way to assist those on their journey to the sacred. Cicely Saunders interpreted end-of-life care as a form of spiritual practice based on Matthew 25 where believers are called to care for the "least of these," the sick, the hungry, the imprisoned, and the stranger. She intentionally chose the name hospice because of its history as a theological concept of care. For Saunders, developing the modern hospice is inseparable from her self-identity as a Christian. Her work with hospice as a physician was a religious vocation in her understanding. My attention to the religious and spiritual identity of the hospice caregiver aligns closely with Saunders view of vocation. I expand on her view of vocation by describing how a theology of hospitality can offer a mode of presence for those in hospice care. In the following section, I turn to the ways a caregiver can apply the theological concept of hospitality to patient encounters as a model that does not require narrative abilities on the part of the patient. Hospitality can be an internal state of being that informs how one views interactions with others, especially those who have nothing to offer us in return. Additionally, hospitality can inform modes of being present with those who are dying as a form of spiritual and religious practice. In the following, I address theological expressions that can be valuable for understanding how hospitality can relate to patient care.

HOSPITALITY AS BEARING WITNESS TO THOSE WHO ARE DYING

The language of witnessing is used to describe intentional, compassionate presence for those at the end of life. Though language of "bearing witness" has a religious history, clinicians also use the term in a medical context to refer to patient-centeredness in the clinical encounter. Arthur Kleinman uses the term "empathic witnessing" when suggesting modes of being present with those who are suffering.[19] Additionally, Rita Charon uses the language of witnessing when discussing what it means to attend closely to patients, listening to them with what Henry James calls "the great empty cup of attention" in a posture of deep listening.[20] Witnessing, or bearing witness, involves continuous presence with a person, offering mindful attention and intentional presence. There is no goal or task involved other than being with the person during their experience.

Cicely Saunders similarly draws on the concept of witnessing when she uses the language "watch with me" as a response to what a patient may desire when the patient faces death.[21] "Watch with me" is what Jesus of Nazareth says the night before his death, knowing that his death is imminent. Even though his death is undertaken freely, he does not want to be alone as he waits for the moment to come. This sense of expectant waiting can also be found with hospice patients who know their time is limited. Not all patients are aware of their environment, many turn inward as they transition to death; yet, the witness can still be present for the individual providing physical comfort through touch as well as providing support for the loved ones of the patient who may need presence and support through their experience of the death.

A value of bearing witness for those transitioning from life is that it does not involve any response from the patient. This is particularly valuable for those patients who may be nonverbal or nonresponsive at the end of life. It is not uncommon for patients to turn inward as they transition, and if those bearing witness understand this, they will not expect any kind of affirmation or acknowledgment of their presence. The dynamic is not one based on mutual recognition or one that is expected to be interactive. There are no expectations that the patient die well or according to the witness's vision or preference. By having no expectations of the patient, one can then honor their intrinsic value as a person of sacred worth, one that does not have to do anything or perform in any way to earn recognition, care, and the presence of another. Cultivating a presence based on hospitality allows a caregiver to continue to be there for patients who may be nonresponsive, agitated, or even combative. There is thus a return to how hospice originally functioned, as a way-station of care for those in need on their way to encounter God, regardless of the condition of the traveler.

ACCOMPANIMENT AS A MODEL OF PRESENCE POSSIBLE REGARDLESS OF NARRATIVE ABILITY

In the works addressed in previous chapters, Ricoeur speaks about the self as embodied, constitutively narrative, and social. In *Living Up to Death*, he offers a way of being present with another person that is centered on receptivity, but not necessarily on the offering or reception of a person's verbal narrative. In this collection of writings, Ricoeur reflects on meaning, care, and presence at the end of life, when one is facing the end of their life. He notes that those who are terminal tend to be life-oriented more than death-oriented—that is, they see themselves as living, not dying.[22] Though they are terminal, they are nevertheless *alive*, and call for being treated accordingly. Using language of "the Essential" to describe transcultural religious awareness, Ricoeur defines compassionate presence as including "the gaze that sees the dying person as still living, as calling on the deepest resources of life, as borne by the emergence of the Essential in [the] experience of still-living. . . . It is the gaze of compassion and not that of the spectator anticipating the already-dead."[23] The gaze of compassion is what defines the act of accompanying for Ricoeur, and it is his language of accompanying that holds value for clinicians and nonprofessional caregivers. Accompanying is a mode of being present for one who is dying—a mode of being that includes an embrace of compassion that holds a person in the present moment rather than being oriented toward the event of the person's death. Accompaniment is informed by narrativity in that it is centered on empathic presence with one who is facing the end of one's narrative. Accompaniment, in this sense, holds great value for caregiver in hospice, in particular.

Through accompanying another, one can be present for and attentive to a patient as a living person and not as merely a dying being or the bearer of diagnosis. Unlike the verbal encounter between caregiver and patient, the act of accompanying can be done with persons who have a cognitive deficit, aphasia or who are unconscious. In these cases it is not the patient's verbal narrative that is interpreted; rather it is their time-narrative that is being interpreted. More clearly, it is the reality that the person is not dead yet, but is living and worthy of compassionate presence that is interpreted. Regarding the physical component of accompanying, in "Prudential Judgment," Ricoeur speaks about the need to maintain the dignity of the patient, noting that "the dignity of the patient is not menaced solely on the level of language, but by all the concessions to familiarity, triviality, [and] vulgarity in the everyday relations between the members of the medical personnel and the hospitalized persons."[24] Similarly, Laurie Zoloth, though she recognizes the place of reflection on one's narrative and the stories present in sacred texts, resists any form of rarefied abstract intellectualism in bioethics that neglects the creatureliness of humans.[25] Dr. Zoloth notes that bioethics does involve rigorous attention to theoretical problems and dilemma/decision-centered consultations, but she says, "Bioethics is also about and perhaps centrally about the tasks of daily living in a fragile body with foreknowledge of our own death."

In *Living Up to Death*, Ricoeur maintains not only the value of physical presence, but also the value of the imagination, linking the imagination to the possibility of compassion and to the ethical domain in medical care. Speaking of the nature of compassion, he writes that, in addition to it having a professional dimension, "there is also a properly ethical dimension, concerning the capacity to accompany in imagination and in sympathy the still living dying person's struggle, still living until dead."[26] He says that act of accompanying and the gaze of compassion are fundamentally relational and more than medical. In other words, nonprofessional caregivers can also be present in an act of accompaniment for the other. The use of narrative method in ethics and in care such as the act of accompanying centers on belief that empathic presence and understanding *is* possible, that the alterity of the other can be overstated. Though there is epistemic distance, there is also empathic connection. Ronald Carson looks to the hyphen as representing the relationship between clinician and patient. He writes, "The hyphenated space in the doctor-patient relationship is a luminal place of ethical encounter, alternating voices and actions—back and forth, address and response. . . . The hyphen points to the prospect of overcoming silence with meaningful conversation."[27]

Relationality between oneself and another is possible even if certainty about the quality of the other's mode of being is not possible to attain. This relationality occurs when the clinician asks for and listens to the narrative offered by the patient. For Ricoeur, the listening involved in accompanying another cannot be considered a merely passive act; rather it is one that can be folded within his understanding of passive activity or active passivity. He uses the language of detachment to describe the act of becoming a vessel for another, service being that which "conjoins the negative detachment (renouncing oneself) and the positive force of detachment, of availability for and openness to the essential."[28] Rita Charon considers the role of detachment as it relates to the empathic imagination when she reflects on the following question: "How does one empty the self or at least suspend the self so as to become a receptive vessel for the language and experience of another? This imaginative, active, receptive, aesthetic experience of donating the self toward the meaning-making of the other is a dramatic, daring, transformative move."[29] This act, the act of listening, appears to be a passive one, but, in fact, it is marked by activity and intentional engagement.[30] One can offer this presence to another through Ricoeur's understanding of the practice of accompanying, regardless of narrative ability on the part of the patient or religious status of the clinician.

Companioning the Dying

Companioning the dying, as described by counselor Greg Yoder, reimagines clinical approaches to patient care for end-of-life caregivers.[31] The companioning model, building on Alan Wofelt's research on grief and mourning and the practices of companioning the bereaved, corresponds with the previous models mentioned, bearing witness and accompaniment, models that demonstrate hospitality to the stranger. Yoder identifies eight aspects of companioning, listed below. Each applies to care for those who might be perceived by clinicians and caregivers as challenging patients, due to cognitive or verbal limits or due to the nature of their pain.

1. Companioning is about honoring all parts of the spirit; it is not about focusing only on intellect.

2. Companioning is more about curiosity; it is less about our expertise.
3. Companioning is about walking alongside; it is less about leading or being led.
4. Companioning the dying is often more about being still; it is not always about urgent movements forward.
5. Companioning the dying means discovering the gifts of sacred silence; it does not mean filling up every moment with talk.
6. Companioning is about being present to another's spiritual and emotional pain; it is not about taking away or fixing it.
7. Companioning is about respecting disorder and confusion; it is not about imposing order and logic.
8. Companioning is about going into the wilderness of the soul with another human being; it is not about thinking you are responsible for finding a way out.[32]

Yoder urges clinicians and caregivers to relax their expectations, often romanticized and frequently self-gratifying, of a rewarding clinical encounter, particularly as such expectations can put pressure on vulnerable patients or family members to labor to please the clinician. Yoder asks that caregivers meet patients where they are, as they are, and critiques scholarship that idealizes the dying experience:

> In much of the literature on dying, there is a glaring lack of reference to spiritually or emotionally distressful deaths that perhaps represent less pleasant examples to teach from. And when they are explored, I get a strong impression that those deaths are viewed as less-than or tragic because the one dying was not able to respond to traditional help or in ways offered by the authors.... The implication is that less poignant, distressful death outcomes, which are many in my experience, are regrettably relegated to the wasn't-that-too-bad category.[33]

Yoder's approach demonstrates hospitality to the stranger by reminding the caregiver that the actual experience of being with patients, unlike the sentimentalized ideal of this experience, can be frustrating, uncomfortable, and shocking rather than peaceful or compelling. To care for a patient expecting that the encounter will be intimate and heartwarming, or even that they will be or comforted by your presence, is unfair to the patient. Such an approach is clinician-centered rather than patient-centered, evincing a reversal of hospitality to the stranger. The practice of companioning the dying, as described by Yoder, addresses the ethical implications of expecting reciprocity or reward from the clinical encounter. Such an approach can lead to the social isolation and potential neglect of patients who challenge the clinician or caregiver.

CONCLUSION

In addition to vocally supporting comprehensive pain management, Cicely Saunders advocated for a form of nonverbal presence with patients who are facing death. She maintained that patients benefit from having someone "be with" them rather than "do for" them, and that patients can be comforted through means that extend beyond the medical. She upheld the intrinsic value of both patients and caregivers in her concept of care: patients do not have to perform what it means to be a model patient and caregivers can serve them by their intentional presence rather than by striving to cure, heal, or fix the patient. Her concept of presence with those who are dying is informed by her Christian faith; however, her model of patient care can be engaged in by those who are secular as the mode of presence does not require any verbal declaration of faith or professional standing as a minister or chaplain.[34] Forms of patient care at the Zen Hospice Project, for instance, recommend similar modes of being with patients.[35] Paul Ricoeur uses the language of accompaniment to describe intentional presence with others, a mode of presence that can be offered by secular caregivers.[36]

Sometimes all it takes is having another person speak to a patient and hold their hand for a patient in terminal distress to be soothed. Patients can present in various ways as they transition to the end of life—some are quiescent and still while others appear physically agitated. Terminal restlessness is a form of agitation that many patients experience as they make the transition toward dying. Terminal restlessness can manifest as physical distress, moaning, picking, clenching one's jaw and limbs, and other forms of physical agitation. Such states are not always assuaged medically; however, a patient may be calmed through the use of touch, soothing words, low lighting, or familiar music. In these instances, the value of a person comfortable with using religious or spiritual modes of comfort cannot be overstated. Currently, doulas for the dying are trained in offering such modes of presence for patients.[37]

Social isolation and the damaging effects such experience has on quality of life for patients can also be addressed through recognition of the value of religious and spiritual forms of behavior. For instance, when patients receive visits by chaplains or volunteers, even if the patient is nonverbal or nonresponsive, the company of another person can still be calming for the patient. Often, it is the caregiver who is uncomfortable with visiting a nonresponsive or agitated patient. This may be because there is an expectation of response or recognition from the patient that the patient is unable to give.

Patients with cognitive or verbal limits do not fit the paradigm of clinician-patient relationality offered by narrative medicine if the encounter depends on conversational reciprocity and understanding. Approached from an expanded perspective, the clinical encounter can be framed as a mode of being with patients without the expectation of narrative satisfaction or dialogical reciprocity, an approach based on the practice of hospitality through bearing witness, accompaniment, and companioning. The value of hospitality is that it does not require anything on the patient's part—there is no expectation of reward or recognition. When one provides care for another as a stranger, it ultimately does not matter whether or not you have access to a patient's thoughts or memories or if they are familiar as the person you knew before. Instead, you care for them in the alien, sometimes radically alien, way they present themselves.

Interacting with a patient with fragmented speech can create discomfort on the part of the visitor. I suggest that in addition to showing the patient hospitality, the experience of internal discomfort is also shown hospitality—one then welcomes the sense of the stranger within. Ricoeur's perspective on the otherness within the self is another way of describing the stranger within one's own person. By learning to be open to feelings of discomfort, a caregiver then will continue to interact with a patient even if the experience is not immediately rewarding. True beneficence then means that a caregiver attends to a patient with no expectation of response on the part of the patient. The patient may not be able to express gratitude, smile, or even make eye contact. Because the grammar of human interaction can involve deeply imbedded, but unspoken expectations, such as the expectation of a response to a question, there can be a high level of discomfort when these expectations go unmet.

An approach informed by religious hospitality is one in which there is no expectation of acknowledgment or reward. Concern is given freely and without conditions. A caregiver approaching a patient in a posture of hospitality makes no demands on the patient, releasing the expectation that the caregiver will experience the satisfaction or stimulation of dialogical reciprocity. Expecting the patient to meet the needs of the caregiver can be a form of objectification. Even with limited dialogical abilities, the patient may be able to intuit that the caregiver is expecting a response from the patient, leading to a state of distress. When a caregiver approaches a patient with no expectation of recognition or reward, the patient is then valued not for his or her ability to perform or satisfy another, but for his or her intrinsic value.

Ricoeur's model of accompaniment, Soelle's model of bearing witness, and Yoder's model of companioning the dying, all offer ways of being with patients that do not require high-level cognition on the patient's part or dialogical encounters based on reciprocity between patients and clinicians. By increasing one's ability to assess and remain present with those who may be experiencing existential distress resulting from life review or the pain of social isolation that can come with aging and cognitive decline, clinicians can give attention to patients' pain in its many dimensions beyond the physical.

NOTES

1. Carlo Leget describes a model of presence with patients that comes from creating "inner space" for their concerns, a model of being with patients that is not explicitly spiritual or religious in nature but nevertheless demonstrates hospitality. *Art of Living, Art of Dying: Spiritual Care for a Good Death* (London: Jessica Kingsley Publishers, 2017).
2. Ricoeur, *Living Up to Death*, 92.
3. Ibid., 94–95.
4. Ibid., 14.
5. Ibid., 15.
6. Ibid., 22.
7. Cicely Saunders, *Watch with Me: Inspiration for a Life in Hospice Care* (Lancaster, UK: Observatory Publications, 2005), 1–2.
8. Selections previously published and reprinted with permission from John Wiley and Sons. Tara Flanagan, "Hospice Care and a Theology for Patients at the End of Life," *Dialog* 53, no. 3 (2014): 259–67.
9. Etymological root is Old French; the Latin is *hospitem*, the nominative Latin is *hospes*.
10. Christine Pohl, *Making Room: Recovering Hospitality as a Christian Tradition* (Grand Rapids, MI: W. B. Eerdmans, 1999), 31.
11. Distinction in the Latin *hospes*, which connotes hosting rather than hospitality.
12. Richard Kearney, *Anatheism: Returning to God after God* (New York: Columbia University Press, 2010).
13. Susan Sontag speaks about the use of this language in her text *Illness as Metaphor* (New York: Vintage Books, 1979).
14. Ira Byock, *Dying Well: Peace and Possibilities at the End of Life* (New York: Riverhead Books, 1998).
15. Dorothee Sölle, *Suffering* (Philadelphia: Fortress Press, 1975).
16. Ibid., 172.
17. Though he has an eschatological vision informed by hope rather than passive resignation and despair, Jürgen Moltmann speaks about the idea of divine suffering to which Soelle refers in his text *The Crucified God: The Cross of Christ as the Foundation and Criticism of Christian Theology* (New York: Harper & Row, 1974).
18. Simone Weil uses the language of loving in the void in her text *Gravity and Grace* (New York: Putnam: 1952).
19. Arthur Kleinman, *The Illness Narratives: Suffering, Healing, and the Human Condition* (New York: Basic Books, 1988), 154.
20. Rita Charon, "Narrative Medicine: Attention, Representation, Affiliation," *Narrative* 13, no. 3 (2005): 261.
21. Cicely Saunders, "'Watch with Me,'" *Nursing Times* 61, no. 48 (1965): 1615.
22. Paul Ricoeur and David Pellauer, *Living Up to Death* (Chicago: University of Chicago Press, 2009), 13–14. The title draws from the first section of the book, the section on which I focus.
23. Ricoeur, *Living Up to Death*, 17.

24. Ricoeur, "Prudential Judgment," 18.

25. Zoloth, "Faith and Reasoning(s)," 270. In a footnote to this claim, she points out that much of the literature in bioethics speaks about the "white, middle-class, university-trained reader," and, because of this, the literature rarely includes accounts from those providing daily care such as nurse's aides or licensed nurses. See note 33.

26. Ricoeur, *Living Up to Death*, 18.

27. Ronald Carson, "The Hyphenated Space: Liminality in the Doctor-Patient Relationship" in *Stories Matter*, 180.

28. Ricoeur, *Living Up to Death*, 51. In this section, Ricoeur is speaking specifically about, in his words, the kenosis/necrosis of Christ, though his words about service parallel his words about accompaniment as receptivity.

29. Charon, "Narrative Medicine," 263.

30. Charon, "Narrative Medicine," 263 from Henry James's *The Wings of a Dove* (London: Mandarin, 1998).

31. Greg Yoder, *Companioning the Dying: A Soulful Guide for Caregivers* (Fort Collins, CO: Companion Press, 2005).

32. Yoder, *Companioning the Dying*.

33. Ibid.

34. Medical sociologist David Clark speaks about the religious roots of hospice care before the Cicely Saunders opened the first formal hospice in 1967. Many hospice practitioners were motivated to care for the dying based on their religious beliefs. See his work "History and Culture in the Rise of Palliative Care" in Sheila Payne, Jane Seymour, and Christine Ingleton's *Palliative Care Nursing: Principles and Evidence for Practice* (Maidenhead: McGraw-Hill International, 2008), 39–54, as well as his biography of Cicely Saunders for details on her background and inspiration to open St. Christopher's Hospice in London. *Cicely Saunders: A Life and Legacy* (New York: Oxford University Press, 2018).

35. Merrill Collett, *At Home with Dying: A Zen Hospice Approach* (Boston: Shambhala, 1999).

36. Paul Ricoeur, *Living Up to Death* (Chicago: University of Chicago Press, 2009).

37. H. Elliot, "Death Doulas Complement Nursing Care at the End of Life," *Nursing Times: NT.* 110, no. 34/35 (2014): 7.

Bibliography

Adams, Carolyn, Julia Bader, and Kathryn Horn. "Timing of Hospice Referral." *Home Health Care Management and Practice* 21, no. 2 (2009): 109–16.
Addis, Donna Rose, and Lynette Tippett. "Memory of Myself: Autobiographical Memory and Identity in Alzheimer's Disease." *Memory* 12, no. 1 (January 2004): 56–74.
Allport, Gordon W. *The Individual and His Religion, a Psychological Interpretation.* New York: Macmillan, 1950.
Allport, Gordon W., and J. Michael Ross. "Personal Religious Orientation and Prejudice." *Journal of Personality and Social Psychology* 5, no. 4 (1967): 432–43.
Anandarajah, G., and E. Hight. "Spirituality and Medical Practice: Using the HOPE Questions as a Practical Tool for Spiritual Assessment." *American Family Physician* 63, no. 1 (January 2001): 81–89.
Ando, Michiyo, Tatsuya Morita, Tatsuo Akechi, and Takuya Okamoto. "Efficacy of Short-Term Life-Review Interviews on the Spiritual Well-being of Terminally Ill Cancer Patients." *Journal of Pain and Symptom Management* 39, no. 6 (2010): 993–1002.
Ando, Michiyo, Tatsuya Morita, and Stephen O'Connor. "Primary Concerns of Advanced Cancer Patients Identified through the Structured Life Review Process: A Qualitative Study using a Text Mining Technique." *Palliative & Supportive Care* 5, no. 3 (2007): 265–71.
Ando, Michiyo, Akira Tsuda, and Tatsuya Morita. "Life Review Interviews on the Spiritual Well-Being of Terminally Ill Cancer Patients." *Supportive Care in Cancer* 15, no. 2 (February 5, 2007): 225–31.
Augustine, Gibb. *The Confessions of Augustine.* New York: Garland Pub., 1980.
Baddeley, A., R. Logie, S. Bressi, S. Della Sala, and H. Spinnler. "Dementia and Working Memory." *The Quarterly Journal of Experimental Psychology* Section A 38, no. 4 (November 1986): 603–18.

Balboni, Michael J., Christina M. Puchalski, and John R. Peteet. "The Relationship between Medicine, Spirituality and Religion: Three Models for Integration." *Journal of Religion and Health* 53, no. 5 (2014): 1586-98.

Barlow, David H. "Unraveling the Mysteries of Anxiety and its Disorders from the Perspective of Emotion Theory." *American Psychologist American Psychologist* 55, no. 11 (2000): 1247-63.

Beauchamp, Tom L., and James F. Childress. *Principles of Biomedical Ethics*. 7th ed. New York: Oxford University Press, 2013.

Berns, Nancy. *Closure: The Rush to End Grief and What It Costs Us*. Philadelphia: Temple University Press, 2011.

Billroth, Theodor, Leon Banov, and Kellogg Speed. *The Medical Sciences in the German Universities: A Study in the History of Civilization*. New York: The Macmillan Company, 1924.

Birren, James E. *Encyclopedia of Gerontology*. Amsterdam; Boston: Academic Press, 2007.

Birren, James E. and Kathryn N. Cochran. *Telling the Stories of Life through Guided Autobiography Groups*. Baltimore: Johns Hopkins University Press, 2001.

Birren, James E. and Donna E. Deutchman. *Guiding Autobiography Groups for Older Adults: Exploring the Fabric of Life*. Baltimore: Johns Hopkins University Press, 1991.

Bishop, Jeffrey Paul. *The Anticipatory Corpse: Medicine, Power, and the Care of the Dying*. Notre Dame, IN: University of Notre Dame Press, 2011.

Bradshaw, A. "The Spiritual Dimension of Hospice: The Secularization of an Ideal." *Social Science & Medicine (1982)* 43, no. 3 (1996): 409-19.

Bramadat, Paul, Harold G. Coward, and Kelli I. Stajduhar. *Spirituality in Hospice Palliative Care*. New York: SUNY Press, 2013.

Branson, Roy. "The Secularization of American Medicine." *The Hastings Center Studies* 1, no. 2 (1973): 17-28.

Bruner, Jerome S. *Actual Minds, Possible Worlds*. Cambridge, MA: Harvard University Press, 1986.

———. *Making Stories: Law, Literature, Life*. New York: Farrar, Straus, and Giroux, 2002.

Buckley, Jenny. *Palliative Care: An Integrated Approach*. Chichester, UK: Wiley-Blackwell, 2008.

Butler, Robert. "The Life Review: An Interpretation of Reminiscence in the Aged." *Psychiatry* 26 (1963): 65-76.

Byock, Ira. *Dying Well: Peace and Possibilities at the End of Life*. New York: Riverhead Books, 1998.

Cadge, Wendy. *Paging God: Religion in the Halls of Medicine*. Chicago; London: The University of Chicago Press, 2012.

Cahill, Lisa Sowle. *Theological Bioethics: Participation, Justice, and Change*. Washington, DC: Georgetown University Press, 2005.

Callahan, Daniel. *False Hopes: Why America's Quest for Perfect Health is a Recipe for Failure*. New York: Simon & Schuster, 1998.

Cassell, Eric J. *The Nature of Suffering: And the Goals of Medicine*. New York: Oxford University Press, 1991.

———. *The Nature of Healing: The Modern Practice of Medicine.* Oxford; New York: Oxford University Press, 2013.
Chambers, Tod. *The Fiction of Bioethics: Cases as Literary Texts.* New York: Routledge, 1999.
Chancellor B., A. Duncan, and A. Chatterjee. "Art Therapy for Alzheimer's Disease and Other Dementias." *Journal of Alzheimer's Disease* 39, no. 1 (2014): 1–11.
Charon, Rita. "The Great Empty Cup of Attention: The Doctor and the Illness in the Wings of the Dove." *Literature and Medicine* 9, no. 1 (1990): 105–24.
———. "Narrative Medicine: Form, Function, and Ethics." *Annals of Internal Medicine* 134, no. 1 (January 2, 2001): 83.
———. "Narrative Medicine: A Model for Empathy, Reflection, Profession, and Trust." *JAMA* 286, no. 15 (October 17, 2001): 1897.
———. "Narrative Medicine: Attention, Representation, Affiliation." *Narrative* 13, no. 3 (2005): 261–70.
———. "A Momentary Watcher, or the Imperiled Reader of 'A Round of Visits.'" *The Henry James Review* 29, no. 3 (2008): 275–86.
———. *Narrative Medicine: Honoring the Stories of Illness.* Oxford: Oxford University Press, 2008.
———. "Narrative Reciprocity." *Hastings Center Report* 44, no. s1 (2014): S21–4.
———. *The Principles and Practice of Narrative Medicine.* New York, NY: Oxford University Press, 2017.
Charon, Rita and Martha Montello. *Stories Matter: The Role of Narrative in Medical Ethics.* New York: Routledge, 2002.
Chochinov, H. M., T. Hack, T. Hassard, L. J. Kristjanson, S. McClement, and M. Harlos. "Dignity Therapy: A Novel Psychotherapeutic Intervention for Patients Near the End of Life." *Journal of Clinical Oncology: Official Journal of the American Society of Clinical Oncology* 23, no. 24 (2005): 5520–25.
Chochinov, Harvey Max. *Dignity Therapy: Final Words for Final Days.* Oxford; New York: Oxford University Press, 2012.
Clark, David. *Cicely Saunders: A Life and Legacy.* Oxford: Oxford University Press USA—OSO, 2018.
Collett, Merrill. *At Home with Dying: A Zen Hospice Approach.* Boston: Shambhala, 1999.
Conway, Kathlyn. *Beyond Words: Illness and the Limits of Expression.* Albuquerque: University of New Mexico Press, 2013.
Coulehan, Jack. "They Wouldn't Pay Attention": Death without Dignity." *American Journal of Hospice and Palliative Medicine* 22, no. 5 (2005): 339–43.
Coulehan, Jack, Peter C. Williams, S. Van McCrary, and Catherine Belling. "The Best Lack All Conviction: Biomedical Ethics, Professionalism, and Social Responsibility." *Cambridge Quarterly of Healthcare Ethics* 12, no. 1 (January 2003): 21–38.
Cutter, William. *Midrash & Medicine: Healing Body and Soul in the Jewish Interpretive Tradition.* 2011.
Crisp, Jane. "Making Sense of the Stories that People with Alzheimer's Tell: A Journey with My Mother." *Nursing Inquiry* 2, no. 3 (1995): 133–40.
Curlin, Farr A. and Peter P. Moschovis. "Is Religious Devotion Relevant to the Doctor-Patient Relationship?" *Journal of Family Practice* 53, no. 8 (2004).

Cutter, William. *Midrash & Medicine: Healing Body and Soul in the Jewish Interpretive Tradition*. Woodstock, VT.: Jewish Lights Pub., 2011.

DasGupta, Sayantani, and Rita Charon. "Personal Illness Narratives: Using Reflective Writing to Teach Empathy:" *Academic Medicine* 79, no. 4 (April 2004): 351–56.

DasGupta, Sayantani, and Marsha Hurst. *Stories of Illness and Healing: Women Write their Bodies*. Kent, OH: Kent State University Press, 2007.

Davis, Dena S., and Laurie Zoloth, eds. *Notes from a Narrow Ridge: Religion and Bioethics*. Hagerstown, MD: University Publishing Group, 1999.

Dees, M. K., M. J. Vernooij-Dassen, W. J. Dekkers, K. C. Vissers, and C. van Weel. "'Unbearable Suffering': A Qualitative Study on the Perspectives of Patients Who Request Assistance in Dying." *Journal of Medical Ethics* 37, no. 12 (2011): 727–34.

De Vries, Raymond, Berlinger, Nancy and Wendy Cadge. *Lost in Translation: The Chaplain's Role in Health Care*. The Hastings Center, 2008.

Dewing, Jan. "Personhood and Dementia: Revisiting Tom Kitwood's Ideas." *OPN International Journal of Older People Nursing* 3, no. 1 (2008): 3–13.

Doeser, M. C., and J. N. Kraay, eds. *Facts and Values: Philosophical Reflections from Western and Non-Western Perspectives*. Martinus Nijhoff Philosophy Library, v. 19. Dordrecht; Boston: M. Nijhoff, 1986.

Doka, Kenneth J. and John B. Breaux. *Living with Grief: Loss in Later Life*. Washington, DC: Hospice Foundation of America, 2002.

DuBose, Edwin R., Ronald P. Hamel, Laurence J. O'Connell, and Park Ridge Center (Ill.), eds. *A Matter of Principles? Ferment in US Bioethics*. Valley Forge, PA: Trinity Press International, 1994.

Duffy, T.P. "The Flexner Report—100 Years Later." *The Yale Journal of Biology and Medicine* 84, no. 3 (2011): 269–76.

Duignan, D., L. Hedley, and R. Milverton. "Exploring Dance as a Therapy for Symptoms and Social Interaction in a Dementia Care Unit." *Nursing Times* 105, no. 30 (2009): 4–17.

Eagly, Alice Hendrickson. *Sex Differences in Social Behavior: A Social-Role Interpretation*. Hillsdale, NJ: L. Erlbaum Associates, 1987.

Edson, Margaret. *Wit: A Play*. New York: Faber and Faber, 1999.

El Haj, Mohamad, Virginie Postal, and Philippe Allaine. "Music Enhances Autobiographical Memory in Mild Alzheimer's Disease." *Educational Gerontology* 38, no. 1 (2012): 30–41.

Elliot, H. "Death Doulas Complement Nursing Care at the End of Life." *Nursing Times* 110, no. 34/35 (2014): 7.

Engel, G.L. "The Need for a New Medical Model: A Challenge for Biomedicine." *Science (New York, NY)* 196, no. 4286 (1977): 129–36.

Engel, John D. *Narrative in Health Care: Healing Patients, Practitioners, Profession, and Community*. Oxford; New York: Radcliffe Publishing, 2008.

Epner, D. E. and W. F. Baile. "Patient-Centered Care: The Key to Cultural Competence." *Annals of Oncology* 23, no. 3 (April 1, 2012): 33–42.

Erikson, Erik H. *The Life Cycle Completed: Extended Version with New Chapters on the Ninth Stage of Development by Joan M. Erikson*. New York: W.W. Norton, 1998.

Evans, Sioned, and Andrew Davison. *Care for the Dying: A Practical and Pastoral Guide* 2014.
Exline, Julie J., Maryjo Prince-Paul, Briana L. Root, Karen S. Peereboom, and Everett L. Worthington. "Forgiveness, Depressive Symptoms, and Communication at the End of Life: A Study with Family Members of Hospice Patients." *Journal of Palliative Medicine* 15, no. 10 (October 2012): 1113–19.
Ferrell, Betty, Shirley Otis-Green, Reverend Pamela Baird, and Andrea Garcia. "Nurses' Responses to Requests for Forgiveness at the End of Life." *Journal of Pain and Symptom Management* 47, no. 3 (2014): 631–41.
Field, Marilyn J., Richard E. Behrman, and Institute of Medicine (US), eds. *When Children Die: Improving Palliative and End-of-Life Care for Children and Their Families*. Washington, DC: National Academy Press, 2003.
Figley, Charles R., ed. *Compassion Fatigue: Coping with Secondary Traumatic Stress Disorder in Those Who Treat the Traumatized*. Brunner/Mazel Psychosocial Stress Series, no. 23. New York: Brunner/Mazel, 1995.
Fishbein, Morris. "The Medical Follies. An Analysis of the Foibles of Some Healing Cults, Including Osteopathy, Homeopathy, Chiropractic, and the Electronic Reactions of Abrams, with Essays on the Antivivisectionists, Health Legislation, Physical Culture, Birth Control and Rejuvenation." *JAMA* 85, no. 19 (November 7, 1925): 1507.
———. *The New Medical Follies: An Encyclopedia of Cultism and Quackery in These United States, with Essays on the Cult of Beauty, the Craze for Reduction, Rejuvenation, Eclecticism, Bread and Dietary Fads, Physical Therapy, and a Forecast as to the Physician of the Future*. New York: AMS Press, 1977.
Fitchett, George. *Assessing Spiritual Needs: A Guide for Caregivers*. Lima, OH: Academic Renewal Press, 2002.
Flaherty, Ellen. "How to Try this: Using Pain-Rating Scales with Older Adults—this Article Examines Three Pain-Rating Scales—the Numeric Rating Scale, the Verbal Descriptor Scale, and the Faces Pain Scale-Revised—that are Widely used with Older Patients." *The American Journal of Nursing* (2008): 40.
Flexner, Abraham and Daniel Updike, Berkeley, Carnegie Foundation for the Advancement of Teaching. Merrymount Press. *Medical Education in the United States and Canada: A Report to the Carnegie Foundation for the Advancement of Teaching*. New York: [s.n.], 1910.
Frank, Arthur W. *The Wounded Storyteller: Body, Illness, and Ethics*. Chicago: University of Chicago Press, 1995.
Frankl, Viktor E. *Man's Search for Meaning: An Introduction to Logotherapy*. New York: Simon & Schuster, 1984.
Friedrich, M.J. "Therapeutic Environmental Design Aims to Help Patients with Alzheimer Disease." *JAMA* 301, no. 23 (June 17, 2009): 243.
Ganguli, Mary, and Eric G. Rodriguez. "Reporting of Dementia on Death Certificates: A Community Study." *Journal of the American Geriatrics Society* 47, no. 7 (July 1999): 842–49.
Gardiner, P. "A Virtue Ethics Approach to Moral Dilemmas in Medicine." *Journal of Medical Ethics* 29, no. 5 (October 1, 2003): 297–302.

Geertz, Clifford. *The Interpretation of Cultures: Selected Essays*. New York: Basic Books, 1973.

Gibson, Faith, and Age Concern (Organization: Great Britain). *Reminiscence and Recall: A Practical Guide to Reminiscence Work*. London: Age Concern, 2006.

Good, Byron. *Medicine, Rationality, and Experience: An Anthropological Perspective*. Cambridge; New York: Cambridge University Press, 1994.

Good, Mary-Jo DelVecchio. *Pain as Human Experience: An Anthropological Perspective*. Berkeley: University of California Press, 1992.

Guéguen, Nicolas, Sebastien Meineri, and Virginie Charles-Sire. "Improving Medication Adherence by Using Practitioner Nonverbal Techniques: A Field Experiment on the Effect of Touch." *Journal of Behavioral Medicine* 33, no. 6 (December 2010): 466–73.

Haber, David. "Life Review: Implementation, Theory, Research, and Therapy." *International Journal of Aging and Human Development* 63, no. 2 (2006): 153–71.

Hahn, Lewis Edwin. *The Philosophy of Paul Ricoeur*. Chicago: Open Court, 1995.

Haight, B. K. "The Therapeutic Role of a Structured Life Review Process in Homebound Elderly Subjects." *Journal of Gerontology* 43, no. 2 (1988): 40–44.

Haight, Barbara K. and Barrett S. Haight. *The Handbook of Structured Life Review*. Baltimore: Health Professions Press, 2007.

Hains, C. A. M. and N. J. Hulbert-Williams. "Attitudes Toward Euthanasia and Physician-Assisted Suicide: A Study of the Multivariate Effects of Healthcare Training, Patient Characteristics, Religion and Locus of Control." *Journal of Medical Ethics* 39, no. 11 (2013): 713–16.

Haker, Hille, "Narrative Ethics in Health Care Chaplaincy," In *Medical Ethics in Health Care Chaplaincy: Essays*, Ed. Walter Moczynski, Hille Haker, and Katrin Bentele (Berlin: Lit, 2009).

Hall, W. David. *Paul Ricoeur and the Poetic Imperative*. Albany, NY: State University of New York Press, 2008.

Handzo, George F., Kevin J. Flannelly, Taryn Kudler, Sarah L. Fogg, Stephen R. Harding, Imam Yusuf H. Hasan, A. Meigs Ross, and Rabbi Bonita E. Taylor. "What Do Chaplains Really Do? II. Interventions in the New York Chaplaincy Study." *Journal of Health Care Chaplaincy* 14, no. 1 (June 10, 2008): 39–56.

Hawkins, Anne Hunsaker. *Reconstructing Illness: Studies in Pathography*. West Lafayette, IN: Purdue University Press, 1993.

Hendricks, Jon. *The Meaning of Reminiscence and Life Review*. Amityville, NY: Baywood Pub. Co., 1995.

Hill, Heather. "Journey without a Map: Dance Therapy with Dementia Patients." *How the Arts make a Difference in Therapy* (1993): 89–105.

Hooyman, Nancy R., and Betty J. Kramer. *Living through Loss: Interventions across the Life Span*. New York: Columbia University Press, 2006.

Howarth, G. "Whatever Happened to Social Class? An Examination of the Neglect of Working Class Cultures in the Sociology of Death." *Health Sociology Review: The Journal of the Health Section of the Australian Sociological Association* 16, no. 5 (2007): 425–35.

Huskey, Rebecca Kathleen. "Paul Ricoeur on Hope: Expecting the Good." *Phenomenology & Literature*, vol. 6. New York: Peter Lang, 2009.

Hyden, L. C. and L. Orulv. "Narrative and Identity in Alzheimer's Disease: A Case Study." *Journal of Aging Studies* 23, no. 4 (2009): 205–14.
Institute for Professionalism Inquiry Conference Proceedings, Rita Charon, Jack Coulehan, and Christina Puchalski. *Toward Healing: Virtuous Practice, Spiritual Care and Narrative Medicine*. Akron, OH: Institute for Professionalism Inquiry, 2005.
James, B. D., S. E. Leurgans, L. E. Hebert, P. A. Scherr, K. Yaffe, and D. A. Bennett. "Contribution of Alzheimer Disease to Mortality in the United States." *Neurology* 82, no. 12 (March 25, 2014): 1045–50.
James, Bryan D. "Dementia From Alzheimer Disease and Mixed Pathologies in the Oldest Old." *JAMA* 307, no. 17 (May 2, 2012): 1798.
James, Henry. *The Portrait of a Lady*. Penguin Classics. London, UK; New York, NY: Penguin Books, 2003.
Johnson, Mark. *Moral Imagination: Implications of Cognitive Science for Ethics*. Chicago: University of Chicago Press, 1997.
Joinson, Carla. "Coping with Compassion Fatigue." *Nursing* 22, no. 4 (April 1992): 116–21.
Jones, Lisa. "Oneself as an Author." *Theory, Culture & Society* 27, no. 5 (September 2010): 49–68.
Jonsen, Albert R. *The Birth of Bioethics*. New York: Oxford University Press, 1998.
Jurecic, Ann. *Illness as Narrative*. Pittsburgh: University of Pittsburgh Press, 2012.
Kearney, Richard. "Narrating Pain: The Power of Catharsis." *Paragraph* 30, no. 1 (2007).
———. *Anatheism: Returning to God After God*. New York: Columbia University Press, 2010.
Kemp, Peter, ed. *Bioethics and Biolaw 1: Judgement of Life*. Copenhagen: Rhodos International Science and Art Publ. & Centre for Ethics and Law, 2000.
Kerr, D. "Mother Mary Aikenhead, the Irish Sisters of Charity and our Lady's Hospice for the Dying." *The American Journal of Hospice & Palliative Care* 10, no. 3 (1993).
Kim, H., M. Chang, K. Rose, and S. Kim. "Predictors of Caregiver Burden in Caregivers of Individuals with Dementia." *Journal of Advanced Nursing* 68, no. 4 (2012): 846–55.
Kindell, Jacqueline, Karen Sage, John Keady, and Ray Wilkinson. "Adapting to Conversation with Semantic Dementia: Using Enactment as a Compensatory Strategy in Everyday Social Interaction." *JLCD International Journal of Language & Communication Disorders* 48, no. 5 (2013): 497–507.
Kitwood, T. M. *Coping with Dementia: The Person Comes First*. Leicester: British Psychological Society, 1996.
Kitwood, Tom. "The Dialectics of Dementia: With Particular Reference to Alzheimer's Disease." *Ageing & Society* 10, no. 2 (1990): 177–96.
Kleinman, Arthur. *The Illness Narratives: Suffering, Healing, and the Human Condition*. New York: Basic Books, 1988.
Kontos, Pia and Gary Naglie. "Expressions of Personhood in Alzheimer's Disease: An Evaluation of Research-Based Theatre as a Pedagogical Tool." *Qualitative Health Research* 17, no. 6 (2007): 799–811.

Kübler-Ross, Elisabeth. *On Death and Dying what the Dying have to Teach Doctors, Nurses, Clergy, and their Own Families.* New York: Macmillan, 1969.

Lawton, M. P., M. Moss, M. H. Kleban, A. Glicksman, and M. Rovine. "A Two-Factor Model of Caregiving Appraisal and Psychological Well-Being." *Journal of Gerontology* 46, no. 4 (July 1, 1991): P181–89.

Leget, Carlo. *Art of Living, Art of Dying: Spiritual Care for a Good Death.* London: Jessica Kingsley Publishers, 2017.

Lepp, Margret, Karin C. Ringsberg, Ann-Kristin Holm, and Gunilla Sellersjö. "Dementia – Involving Patients and their Caregivers in a Drama Programme: The Caregivers' Experiences." *JOCN Journal of Clinical Nursing* 12, no. 6 (2003): 873–81.

Levin, J. S. "Religion and Spirituality in Medicine: Research and Education." *JAMA* 278, no. 9 (September 3, 1997): 792–93.

Lewis, M. I. and R. N. Butler. "Life-Review Therapy. Putting Memories to Work in Individual and Group Psychotherapy." *Geriatrics* 29, no. 11 (1974): 165–73.

Lewis, Milton James. *Medicine and Care of the Dying: A Modern History.* Oxford; New York: Oxford University Press, 2007.

Lindemann, Hilde. *Damaged Identities, Narrative Repair.* Ithaca, NY: Cornell University Press, 2001.

Lorde, Audre. *The Cancer Journals.* San Francisco: Aunt Lute Books, 1997.

Lysaught, Therese. "Respect: Or, How Respect for Persons Became Respect for Autonomy." *The Journal of Medicine and Philosophy* 29, no. 6 (2004): 665–80.

———. *On Moral Medicine: Theological Perspectives in Medical Ethics.* Grand Rapids, MI: W. B. Eerdmans Pub. Co., 2012.

MacIntyre, Alasdair C. *After Virtue: A Study in Moral Theory.* Notre Dame, IN: University of Notre Dame Press, 1981.

MacIntyre, Alisdair, and The Hegeler Institute. "Epistemological Crises, Dramatic Narrative and the Philosophy of Science:" Edited by Sherwood J. B. Sugden. *Monist* 60, no. 4 (1977): 453–72.

Mako, Caterina, Kathleen Galek, and Shannon R. Poppito. "Spiritual Pain among Patients with Advanced Cancer in Palliative Care." *Journal of Palliative Medicine* 9, no. 5 (October 2006): 1106–13.

Maleske, M. "Hospice Care. Pet Therapy." *Hospitals & Health Networks/AHA* 78, no. 11 (2004).

Mattingly, Cheryl. *Healing Dramas and Clinical Plots: The Narrative Structure of Experience.* Cambridge Studies in Medical Anthropology 7. Cambridge, UK; New York, NY: Cambridge University Press, 1998.

Maugans, T. A. "The SPIRITual History." *Archives of Family Medicine* 5, no. 1 (January 1, 1996): 11–16.

Mastel-Smith, B., B. Binder, A. Malecha, G. Hersch, L. Symes, and J. McFarlane. "Testing Therapeutic Life Review Offered by Home Care Workers to Decrease Depression among Home-Dwelling Older Women." *Issues in Mental Health Nursing* 27, no. 10 (2006): 1037–49.

Meier, Diane E. "Palliative Care in Hospitals." *JHM Journal of Hospital Medicine* 1, no. 1 (2006): 21–28.

Miller, Susan C., Pedro Gozalo, and Vincent Mor. "Hospice Enrollment and Hospitalization of Dying Nursing Home Patients." *The American Journal of Medicine* 111, no. 1 (2001): 38.
Mitchell, Susan L., Susan C. Miller, Joan M. Teno, Dan K. Kiely, Roger B. Davis, and Michele L. Shaffer. "Prediction of 6-Month Survival of Nursing Home Residents With Advanced Dementia Using ADEPT vs Hospice Eligibility Guidelines." *JAMA* 304, no. 17 (November 3, 2010): 1929.
Moczynski, Walter, ed. *Medical Ethics in Health Care Chaplaincy: Essays. Medical Ethics in Health Care Chaplaincy*. Berlin: Lit, 2009.
Mohrmann, Margaret E. "Ethical Grounding for a Profession of Hospital Chaplaincy." *The Hastings Center Report* 38, no. 6 (2008): 18–23.
Moltmann, Jürgen. *The Crucified God: The Cross of Christ as the Foundation and Criticism of Christian Theology*. 1st US ed. New York: Harper & Row, 1974.
Monroe, Barbara and David Oliviere. *Patient Participation in Palliative Care: A Voice for the Voiceless*. New York: Oxford University Press, 2003.
Montgomery, Kathryn. *Doctors' Stories: The Narrative Structure of Medical Knowledge*. Princeton, NJ: Princeton University Press, 1991.
———. *How Doctors Think: Clinical Judgment and the Practice of Medicine*. Oxford; New York: Oxford University Press, 2006.
Najjar, Nadine, Louanne W. Davis, Kathleen Beck-Coon, and Caroline Carney Doebbeling. "Compassion Fatigue: A Review of the Research to Date and Relevance to Cancer-Care Providers." *Journal of Health Psychology* 14, no. 2 (March 2009): 267–77.
Neimeyer, Robert A. *Techniques of Grief Therapy: Creative Practices for Counseling the Bereaved*. New York: Routledge, 2012.
Noll, Mark A. *A History of Christianity in the United States and Canada*. Grand Rapids, MI: W. B. Eerdmans, 1992.
Normann, Hans Ketil, Astrid Norberg, and Kenneth Asplund. "Confirmation and Lucidity during Conversations with a Woman with Severe Dementia." *Journal of Advanced Nursing* 39, no. 4 (August 2002): 370–76.
Nussbaum, Martha Craven. *Love's Knowledge: Essays on Philosophy and Literature*. New York: Oxford University Press, 1990.
———. *The Fragility of Goodness: Luck and Ethics in Greek Tragedy and Philosophy*. Rev. ed. Cambridge, UK; New York: Cambridge University Press, 2001.
O' Mahony, S. "Against Narrative Medicine." *Perspectives in Biology and Medicine* 56, no. 4 (2013): 611–19.
Ong, Chi-Keong and Duncan Forbes. "Embracing Cicely Saunders's Concept of Total Pain." *BMJ: British Medical Journal* 331, no. 7516 (2005): 576–77.
Örulv, Linda, Hydén and Lars-Christer. "Confabulation: Sense-Making, Self-Making and World-Making in Dementia." *Discourse Studies* 8, no. 5 (2006): 647–73.
Parsons, Talcott. "The Sick Role and the Role of the Physician Reconsidered." *The Milbank Memorial Fund Quarterly. Health and Society* 53, no. 3 (1975): 257–78.
Payne, Sheila. *Palliative Care Nursing Principles and Evidence for Practice*. Maidenhead: Open University Press, 2009.

Phelan, James. "Editor's Column: Who's Here? Thoughts on Narrative Identity and Narrative Imperialism." *Narrative* 13, no. 3 (2005): 205–10.

Pohl, Christine D. *Making Room: Recovering Hospitality as a Christian Tradition.* Grand Rapids, MI: W. B. Eerdmans, 1999.

Polubinski, Joseph P., and Laurie West. "Implementation of a Massage Therapy Program in the Home Hospice Setting." *Journal of Pain and Symptom Management* 30, no. 1 (July 2005): 104–6.

Puchalski, Christina. "The Role of Spirituality in Health Care." *Proceedings (Baylor University. Medical Center)* 14, no. 4 (2001): 352–57.

———. "Spirituality and Medicine: Curricula in Medical Education." *Journal of Cancer Education* 21, no. 1 (March 1, 2006): 14–18.

———. "Spiritual Issues as an Essential Element of Quality Palliative Care: A Commentary." *The Journal of Clinical Ethics* 19, no. 2 (2008): 160–62.

Puchalski, Christina, and Anna L. Romer. "Taking a Spiritual History Allows Clinicians to Understand Patients More Fully." *Journal of Palliative Medicine* 3, no. 1 (March 2000): 129–37.

Puchalski, Christina M. and David B. Larson. "Developing Curricula in Spirituality and Medicine." *Academic Medicine* 73, no. 9 (1998): 970–74.

Rahner, Karl. *Foundations of Christian Faith: An Introduction to the Idea of Christianity.* New York: Seabury Press, 1978.

Ramsey, Paul. *The Patient as Person: Explorations in Medical Ethics.* New Haven: Yale University Press, 1970.

Randall, William. "Storywork: Autobiographical Learning in Later Life." *ACE New Directions for Adult and Continuing Education* 2010, no. 126 (2010): 25–36.

Rando, Therese. "An Investigation of Grief and Adaptation in Parents Whose Children Have Died from Cancer." *Journal of Pediatric Psychology* 8, no. 1 (1983): 3–20.

Reisberg, Barry, Steven H. Ferris, Mony J. de Leon, Elia Sinaiko Emile Franssen, Alan Kluger, Pervez Mir, Jeffrey Borenstein, Ajax E. George, Emma Shulman, Gertrude Steinberg, and Jacob Cohen. "Stage-Specific Behavioral, Cognitive, and in Vivo Changes in Community Residing Subjects with Age-Associated Memory Impairment and Primary Degenerative Dementia of the Alzheimer Type." *DDR Drug Development Research* 15, nos. 2–3 (1988): 101–14.

Reverby, Susan. *Examining Tuskegee: The Infamous Syphilis Study and its Legacy.* Chapel Hill: University of North Carolina Press, 2009.

Richmond, Caroline. "Dame Cicely Saunders." *BMJ: British Medical Journal* 331, no. 7510 (2005): 238.

Ricoeur, Paul. *The Symbolism of Evil.* New York: Harper & Row, 1967.

———. *Time and Narrative.* Chicago: University of Chicago Press, 1984.

———. *Fallible Man.* New York: Fordham University Press, 1986.

———. *Oneself as Another.* Chicago: University of Chicago Press, 1992.

———. *Memory, History, Forgetting.* Chicago: University of Chicago Press, 2004.

———. *Living Up to Death.* Translated by David Pellauer. University of Chicago Press, 2009.

Rodriquez, J. "Narrating Dementia: Self and Community in an Online Forum." *Qualitative Health Research* 23, no. 9 (2013): 1215–27.

Saunders, Cicely. "Watch with Me." *Nursing Times* 61, no. 48 (1965): 1615–17.
———. *St. Christopher's in Celebration: Twenty-One Years at Britain's First Modern Hospice*. London: Hodder and Stoughton, 1988.
———. "St Christopher's Hospice." *St Thomas' Hospital Gazette* (1991): 10–14.
———. *Cicely Saunders: Selected Writings 1958–2004*. Oxford; New York: Oxford University Press, 2006.
Saunders, Cicely M. and Mary Baines. *Living with Dying: The Management of Terminal Disease*. Oxford; New York: Oxford University Press, 1983.
Saunders, Cicely M., Mary Baines, and R. J. Dunlop. *Living with Dying: A Guide to Palliative Care*. Oxford; New York: Oxford University Press, 1995.
Saunders, Cicely M., and David Clark. *Cicely Saunders: Founder of the Hospice Movement: Selected Letters 1959–1999*. Oxford: Clarendon, 2002.
Scarry, Elaine. *The Body in Pain: The Making and Unmaking of the World*. New York: Oxford University Press, 1985.
Shanafelt, Tait D. "Enhancing Meaning in Work: A Prescription for Preventing Physician Burnout and Promoting Patient-Centered Care." *JAMA* 302, no. 12 (September 23, 2009): 1338.
Siebold, Cathy. *The Hospice Movement: Easing Death's Pains*. New York; Toronto; New York: Twayne; Maxwell Macmillan Canada; Maxwell Macmillan International, 1992.
Smith, Glenn E. and Mark W. Bondi. *Mild Cognitive Impairment and Dementia: Definitions, Diagnosis, and Treatment*. New York: Oxford University Press, 2013.
Sölle, Dorothee. *Suffering*. Philadelphia: Fortress Press, 1975.
Stagno, Susan, and Michael Blackie. *From Reading to Healing: Teaching Medical Professionalism Through Literature* Kent, OH: Kent State University Press, 2019.
Strawson, Galen. "Against Narrativity." *Ratio* 17, no. 4 (2004): 428–52.
Sontag, Susan, and Susan Sontag. *Illness as Metaphor; and, AIDS and Its Metaphors*. 1st Anchor Books ed. New York: Doubleday, 1990.
Spiro, Howard, Mary G. McCrea Curnen, Enid Peschel, and Deborah St. James. *Empathy and the Practice of Medicine: Beyond Pills and the Scalpel*. New Haven: Yale University Press, 1996
Sulmasy, Daniel. *The Rebirth of the Clinic: An Introduction to Spirituality in Health Care*. Washington, DC: Georgetown University Press, 2006.
———. "Spiritual Issues in the Care of Dying Patients: '. . . It's Okay between Me and God'." *JAMA* 296, no. 11 (2006): 1385–92.
———. "Spirituality, Religion, and Clinical Care." *Chest* 135, no. 6 (2009): 1634–42.
———. "Ethos, Mythos, and Thanatos: Spirituality and Ethics at the End of Life." *Journal of Pain and Symptom Management* 46, no. 3 (2013): 447–51.
Sweeting, Helen and Mary Gilhooly. "Dementia and the Phenomenon of Social Death." *Sociology of Health & Illness* 19, no. 1 (1997): 93–117.
Swinton, John and Richard Payne. "Living Well and Dying Faithfully: Christian Practices for End-of-Life Care." Grand Rapids, MI: W. B. Eerdmans Pub. Co., 2009.
Tappen, Ruth M., Christine Williams, Sarah Fishman, and Theris Touhy. "Persistence of Self in Advanced Alzheimer's Disease." *Image: The Journal of Nursing Scholarship* 31, no. 2 (June 1999): 121–25.

Teilhard de Chardin, Pierre. *The Divine Milieu; an Essay on the Interior Life.* New York: Harper, 1960.

Thompson, Teresa L. *Handbook of Health Communication.* New York, NY: Routledge, 2008.

———. "The Applicability of Narrative Ethics." *Journal of Applied Communication Research* 37, no. 2 (May 2009): 188–95.

Tillich, Paul. *The Courage to Be.* New Haven, CT: Yale University Press, 1952.

Timmer, E., G. J. Westerhof, and F. Dittmann-Kohli. "'When Looking Back on My Past Life I Regret...': Retrospective Regret in the Second Half of Life." *Death Studies* 29, no. 7 (2005): 625–44.

Tolstoy, Leo, Lynn Solotaroff. *The Death of Ivan Illyich.* Toronto; New York: Bantam Books, 1985.

Trevino, K. M., M. Balboni, A. Zollfrank, T. Balboni, and H. G. Prigerson. "Negative Religious Coping as a Correlate of Suicidal Ideation in Patients with Advanced Cancer." *Psycho-Oncology* 23, no. 8 (2014): 936–45.

Turner, John C. *Rediscovering the Social Group: Self-Categorization Theory.* Oxford, UK; New York, NY: B. Blackwell, 1987.

Wald, Florence S. and Judith L. Lief. Yale University, School of Nursing. "In Quest of the Spiritual Component of Care for the Terminally Ill: Proceedings of a Colloquium May 3–4, 1986, Yale University School of Nursing." [publisher not identified], 1986.

Ware, Bronnie. *The Top Five Regrets of the Dying: A Life Transformed by the Dearly Departing.* 1st ed. Carlsbad, CA: Hay House, 2012.

Webster, Jeffrey Dean and Mary E. McCall. "Reminiscence Functions Across Adulthood: A Replication and Extension." *Journal of Adult Development* 6, no. 1 (1999): 73–85.

Weil, Simone. *Gravity and Grace.* London: Routledge and K. Paul, 1972.

White, Michael and David Epston. *Narrative Means to Therapeutic Ends.* New York: Norton, 1990.

Wolfelt, Alan. *Companioning the Bereaved: A Soulful Guide for Caregivers.* Fort Collins, CO: Companion, 2006.

Wray, Alison. "Formulaic Language as a Barrier to Effective Communication with People with Alzheimer's Disease." *CMLR Canadian Modern Language Review/La Revue Canadienne Des Langues Vivantes* 67, no. 4 (2011): 429–58.

Yaffe, Kristine. "Treatment of Alzheimer Disease and Prognosis of Dementia: Time to Translate Research to Results." *JAMA* 304, no. 17 (November 3, 2010): 1952.

Yoder, Greg. *Companioning the Dying: A Soulful Guide for Caregivers.* Fort Collins, CO: Companion Press, 2012.

Zalaquett, Carlos P. and Andrea N. Stens. "Psychosocial Treatments for Major Depression and Dysthymia in Older Adults: A Review of the Research Literature." *Journal of Counseling & Development* 84, no. 2 (2006): 192–201.

Zaner, R. M. "Medicine and Dialogue." *The Journal of Medicine and Philosophy* 15, no. 3 (1990): 303–25.

Index

accompaniment model, 119–21, 123; companioning the dying, 121–22; Ricoeur, Paul, 119–21
acute-care environment, 98
AD. *See* Alzheimer's disease (AD)
agent narrativity, 88. *See also* partial narrativity; social narrativity; moral identity for, 88–90
"Alexithymia," 18
Allport, Gordon: *Individual and His Religion, The,* 49
Alzheimer's disease (AD), 84–87, 96, 103n11; patients: (assisted recall, 92, 93; confabulation, 91; language ability, 91; moral analysis, 90)
Andiman, Ronald: "Midrash and Medicine," 18
Aristotle, 8–9, 33; *Poetics,* 9, 70
art therapy, 92–93, 101
assisted recall, 92–93
Augustine, Gibb, 72; *Confessions,* 72
autobiography, 65, 66
autonomy, 15, 16

Balint, Michael, 5
bearing witness, 121; hospitality, 118–19; Soelle, Dorothee, 117–19, 124
Belmont Report, 6, 23n36
bereavement care, 55n30, 94, 99

bioethics, 6–7, 12, 13, 120
Booth, Wayne, 10, 15, 25n54
Brody, Howard, 15
Bruner, Jerome, 5, 94
Butler, Judith, 18
Butler, Robert, 67–69, 85, 96
Byock, Ira, 35, 71, 115

Cancer Journals, The (Lorde), 65
caregivers, hospitality practice and, 112–15
Carson, Ronald, 121
Cassell, Eric, 6–7, 18, 19
certainty, 16
Chambers, Tod, 16; *Fiction of Bioethics, The,* 7–8
chaplains, 44, 45, 51–52, 93; and life review, 39–41; role, 41–43
Charon, Rita, 4, 6–8, 10, 15–18, 59, 95, 118, 121; narrative competence, 17, 18; parallel charting for clinicians, 17; *Stories Matter* and *Narrative Medicine,* 17; virtue ethics, 17
Chochinov, Harvey, 64
clinical caregivers, 42
clinical detachment, 3–4, 19
clinical empathy, 4
clinical medical education, religion in, 48

clinical pastoral education (CPE), 43–44
clinical pedagogy, 8; critique, 15
clinical practice, 14–20
clinical reasoning, narrativity in, 19
clinical training, benefits of, 17
clinicians: narrative knowledge, 10; narrative methods, 8–11; practice, 7–8
cognitive decline, 84–87, 101
cognitive impairment, 84
cognitively compromised patients, 87–88
companioning the dying: Yoder, Greg, 121–22, 124
compassion fatigue, 22n13
condemnation, 36
confabulation, 84; partial narrativity, 91–92
Confessions (Augustine), 72
Connelly, Julia, 10, 25n55
Conway, Kathlyn, 19–20
Coulehan, Jack, 3–4, 86
CPE. *See* clinical pastoral education (CPE)
Crisp, Jane, 91

DasGupta, Sayantani: *Stories of Illness and Healing*, 4
Death of Ivan Ilyich, The (Edson and Tolstoy), 25n54, 70–72
dementia, 84–86, 102n1; social enactment, 87
dementia patients: assisted recall, 92; language ability, 91; loss of socialization, 85–86
denial of illness, 114
desire for forgiveness, 71–72
detachment, 121
Dignity Therapy, 64
dying: hospitality as bearing witness, 118–19; meditation, 108–11

EBM. *See* evidence-based medicine (EBM)
emotional distress, 40–42, 44

emotional pain, 36, 37, 39, 40, 110, 115
emotional stress, 38
empathic awareness, 9, 10
empathic presence, 8
empathic witnessing, 118
emplotment, 11, 14
end of life, meditation, on, 108–11
end-of-life patients: desire for forgiveness, 71–72; grief over lost time, 72–73; life review, 61–63; moral self-reflection, 71; regret, 69–71
Engel, George, 5
Erikson, Erik, 69
ethical analysis, life review: desire for forgiveness, 71–72; grief over lost time, 72–73; regret, 69–71
ethical intention, 33
ethical self, 73
ethical self-analysis, 70, 72; religion, 69
ethics, 120
evidence-based medicine (EBM), 2, 21n5, 42
existential distress, 40–42, 44, 72
existential pain, 42
extrinsic religiosity, 49

familiar texts, 93–94
feeling of meaninglessness, 71
FICA, 46, 49, 51
Fiction of Bioethics, The (Chambers), 7–8
Fishbein, Morris, 2
Flanagan, John, 24n40
Flexner, Abraham: medical education reform, 1–2
Fragility of Goodness, The (Nussbaum), 9
Frank, Arthur, 6, 15, 19–20; *Wounded Storyteller, The*, 66

gaze of compassion, 119–20
Geertz, Clifford, 5
Goldenstein, Catherine, 108
Good, Byron, 5

Good, Mary Jo Delvecchio, 5
grief over lost time, 72–73
guided autobiography, 64–65

Hall, David, 13, 25n64, 26n74
Hawkins, Anne Hunsaker, 5
health, WHO definition of, 46
hermeneutical approach, 10–11, 15, 16
Holmes, Sherlock, 19
home care, 96–97. *See also* hospital care
Hooyman, N., 45
HOPE, 49, 51
hospice caregivers, theology of hospitality for, 113, 117–18
hospice care model, 53, 96, 99; life review and narrative practices, 39; (bereavement care, 44–46; chaplains and, 39–41; clinical pastoral education, 43–44; role of chaplain, 41–43; social selfhood, 45; spiritual counselors, 39–41); life review in moral reflection, 67–69; limits, 98; narrative identity, 100; and palliative care models, 60; patient identity, 33–35; (pain and, 36–38); religious dimension of human experience, 46–48; Saunders, Cicely, 33–36, 118; spiritual assessments and life review, 51–53; total pain, 35–36
hospital care, 97–98
hospitality, 124; as bearing witness, 118–19; hospice patients and caregivers, 112–15; origin of the word, 111–12; theology, 113, 117–18
hostility, 113–14
hosting pain, 114–15
human experience, religious dimension of, 46–48
human value, 49, 50
Huskey, Rebecca, 26
Hyden, Lars-Christer, 87

Illness as Narrative (Jurecic), 52
illness narratives, 4–6, 19, 65–66
impaired ability, 84–87

imputation capability, 75
Individual and His Religion, The (Allport), 49
individualism, 86–87
intrinsic religiosity, 49
inward pain, 36
isolation, 38

James, Henry, 7, 118; *Portrait of a Lady,* 9
James, William, 49
JCAHO. *See* Joint Commission on Accreditation of Healthcare Organizations (JCAHO)
Johnson, Mark, 8
Joint Commission on Accreditation of Healthcare Organizations (JCAHO), 43, 46, 52
Jones, Anne Hudson, 17
Jones, Lisa, 12
Journal of the American Medical Association, 2
Jurecic, Ann, 4; *Illness as Narrative,* 52

Kearney, Richard, 113, 117
Kleinman, Arthur, 5, 65, 118
Kramer, B., 45

Levinas, Emmanuel, 18, 33
Lewis, Milton, 68
life and death, 49
"Life: A Story in Search of a Narrator" (Ricoeur), 11
life expectancy, 84, 102n4
life plan, limits of, 73–75
life review, 38, 59–60, 70, 111–12; Alzheimer's disease and, 84–85; capabilities necessary for, 66–67; dialogical process, 40; differences between other modalities and, 66; Dignity Therapy, 64; end-of-life patients, 61–63; ethical analysis: (desire for forgiveness, 71–72; grief over lost time, 72–73; regret, 69–71); guided autobiography,

64–65; hospice as mode of moral reflection, 67–69; illness narratives, 65–66; limits of Ricoeur's life plan, 73–75; moral identity and, 87–88, 99; narrative practices, hospice care, 39; (bereavement care, 44–46; chaplains, 39–41; clinical pastoral education, 43–44; role of chaplain, 41–43; social selfhood, 45; spiritual counselors, 39–41); reminiscence versus, 62–63; spiritual assessments, 51–53
listening, 121
Living Up to Death (Ricoeur), 33, 108, 109, 119, 120
Living with Dying: The Management of Terminal Disease (Saunders), 33
loneliness, 38
long-term residential care, 96, 98–99
Lorde, Audre: *Cancer Journals, The,* 65
Lost in Translation: The Chaplain's Role in Health Care (de Vries, Berlinger and Cadge), 42

MacIntyre, Alasdair, 5, 6, 32
Mattingly, Cheryl, 5
medical education reform, 1–2
medical ethics, 6, 14–20; principlism, 50
medical humanities, narrative in, 4–7
Medicare, 41, 98; guidelines, 41, 44–45
meditation, on end of life, 108–11
memory loss, 85
"Midrash and Medicine" (Andiman), 18
Miller, Larry, 19
mimesis, 11–13, 19
"mirror-gazing," 68
Mohrmann, Margaret, 52
Montgomery, Kathryn, 16
moral identity, 99–100; agent narrativity, 88–90; life review, 87–88
moral reflection, life review in hospice and, 67–69
moral self-evaluation, 112
motor function decline, 84

music therapy, 92–93

narrative and medical humanities, 4–7
narrative ability and accompaniment model, 119–22
narrative competence, 10, 17, 18
narrative ethics, 13, 15
narrative identity, 14, 32–33, 74–75; clinical encounter, 99–100; long-term residential care and, 98–99; social narrativity, 94–95
narrative medicine: clinical pastoral education, 43–44; defined, 7; individualism, 86–87; limits, 95
narrative methods, 8–11, 40–41; religion and limits, 111–12
narrative practice: context of care effects, 95–96; (home care, 96–97; hospital care, 97–98); spiritual assessments, 48–53
narrative self, 11–14, 16, 18, 97
"narratives of triumph," 19–20
narrativity, 15, 16, 18; concept, 19
Nelson, Hilde Lindemann, 10, 15
non-acute care contexts, 98
non-reflective professionalism, 3
nonverbal patients, religion and, 111–12
Nussbaum, Martha, 15, 27n86; *Fragility of Goodness, The,* 9

Oneself as Another (Ricoeur), 13, 15, 26n74, 28n89, 31–33, 54n7, 75
Orulv, Linda, 87

pain, 52, 112–15; control, 35; of despair, 36; emotional, 36, 37, 39, 40, 110, 115; loneliness, 38; management, 34–36, 45; patient identity, 36–38; physical, 36, 37, 39–40, 71, 115; social, 36, 37, 39, 40, 42, 73, 110; spiritual, 36, 37, 39, 40, 42, 71, 73, 115; total, 35–36, 38, 39, 70, 110, 114
palliative care models, 60

Parkinson's disease, 84, 96. *See also* Alzheimer's disease (AD)
partial narrativity, 90; assisted recall, 92–93; confabulation as, 91–92; use of familiar texts, 93–94
passivity, 12, 32
pastoral care, 100
patient identity, 117; hospice model of care, 33–35; pain, 36–38; religious, 46–51; spiritual, 46, 48–51
patient's abilities, limitations, 84–87
patient's recognition, 46
Pellegrino, Edward, 6
physical pain, 36, 37, 39–40, 71, 115
physician and patient relationship, 13
Poetics (Aristotle), 9, 70
Portrait of a Lady (James), 9
practice of clinicians, 7–8
prayer, 41
principlism, 12, 14–16, 50
"Prudential Judgment, Deontological Judgment and Reflexive Judgment in Medical Ethics" (Ricouer), 13, 120
psalmic language, 116
Puchalski, Christine, 4, 46–48, 52–53, 98

quality-of-life measures, 24n40

Rahner, Karl, 68
Ramsey, Paul, 6, 14
real-time narration, 93
recounting capability, 74
regret, 68–71
relationality, 121
religion: clinical medical education, 48; limiting the narrative methods, 111–12; and spirituality, 46–51
religiosity, 47, 49–50
religious care, 41–42
religious dimension of human experience, 46–48
religious hospitality, 124
religious identity, 46, 48–51, 112; hospice caregiver, 117–18

Religious Orientation Scale, 49
reminiscence versus life review, 62–63
"restitution narratives," 20
Ricoeur, Paul, 5, 6, 8, 9, 19, 26n64, 42, 101; accompaniment model, 119–21, 123, 124; dialectic of sameness-variability, 31–32; hermeneutical approach, 10–11, 15; "Life: A Story in Search of a Narrator," 11; limits of life plan concept, 73–75; *Living Up to Death,* 33, 108, 109, 119–20; meditation on end of life, 108–11; mimesis, 11–13, 19; narrative identity, 32–33; narrative self, 11–14; *Oneself as Another,* 13, 15, 26n74, 28n89, 31–33, 54n7, 75; otherness perspective, 124; "Prudential Judgment, Deontological Judgment and Reflexive Judgment in Medical Ethics," 13, 120; "Self and the Ethical Aim, The," 33; selfhood, 31–32, 38, 45, 54, 74–75; *Time and Narrative,* 11, 13, 15, 31
Rogers, Carl, 5
Ross, Michael, 49

Saunders, Cicely, 33, 109, 111; definition of pain, 34; end-of-life care, 118; feelings of regret, 71; hospice care model, 33–36, 118; *Living with Dying: The Management of Terminal Disease,* 33; physical pain, 40; social pain, 73; spiritual identity, 48; spiritual pain, 39, 73; total pain concept, 35–36, 38, 39, 70, 110, 114; *Watch with Me,* 110, 118; witnessing concept, 118
Scarry, Elaine, 52
scrapbooks, 92
"Self and the Ethical Aim, The" (Ricoeur), 33
self-awareness, 18
self-blame, 36
selfhood, 12, 13, 31–32, 38, 45, 54, 74–75, 90, 111–12, 116

short-term life review, 67
social enactment, 87
social gatherings, 93
social isolation, 63, 122, 123
social media, 93
social narrativity, 94–95, 101; benefit, 95
social pain, 36, 37, 39, 40, 42, 73, 110
social selfhood, 45
Soelle, Dorothee, 107, 124; bearing witness, 117–19, 124; suffering, 115–16; theological orientation, 116
solicitude, 73
SPIRIT, 49, 51
spiritual assessments, 111–12; critiques, 50–51; life review and, 51–53; as narrative practice, 48–50
spiritual care, 41–42
spiritual counselors and life review, 39–41
spiritual distress, 38, 40–41, 47
spiritual identity, 46, 48–51; hospice caregiver, 117–18
spirituality, religion and, 46–51
spiritual pain, 36, 37, 39, 40, 42, 71, 73, 115
Spiro, Howard, 17
Stories of Illness and Healing (DasGupta), 4
Strawson, Galen, 67, 74
suffering, 115–16
Sulmasy, Daniel, 46–48, 52, 70

Tartaglia, Alexander, 44
Tasma, David (patient), 110
terminal restlessness, 123
theology of hospitality, 113, 117–18
therapeutic environmental design, 85
Thomas, Dylan, 114
Tillich, Paul, 68
Time and Narrative (Ricoeur), 11, 13, 15, 31
total pain, 35–36, 38, 39, 70, 110, 114
Turner, John, 89

value of care and healing, 7
verbally compromised patients, 87–88
video, 92
virtue ethics, 17

Ware, Bonnie, 70
Watch with Me (Saunders), 110, 118
Weil, Simone, 116
well-being, 7
Witness Protection Program, 97
Wofelt, Alan, 121
World Health Organization, 46
Wounded Storyteller, The (Frank), 66

Yoder, Greg, 108; companioning the dying, 121–22, 124

Zaner, Richard, 5
Zoloth, Laurie, 16, 120

About the Author

Tara Flanagan, PhD, is assistant professor of religious studies at Maria College in Albany, NY. She also holds a clinical appointment as hospice chaplain at New York-Presbyterian/Jansen Hospice and Palliative Care. Her research centers on religion, medicine, and ethics with special attention given to religious and spiritual care for patients and families in hospice and the role of health-care chaplains in the clinical encounter.

www.ingramcontent.com/pod-product-compliance
Lightning Source LLC
Chambersburg PA
CBHW020125010526
44115CB00008B/980